NATURAL
ALTERNATIVES
TO VIOXX, CELEBREX
& other Anti-Inflammatory
Prescription Drugs

SECOND EDITION

Carol Simontacchi

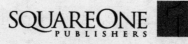

SQUAREONE
PUBLISHERS

COVER DESIGNER: Jacqueline Michelus
IN-HOUSE EDITOR: Joanne Abrams
TYPESETTER: Gary A. Rosenberg

Square One Publishers
115 Herricks Road
Garden City Park, NY 11040
516-535-2010 • 877-900-BOOK
www.squareonepublishers.com

CONTENTS

For my four daughters,
who give me so much pleasure
(and very little pain),
and my fifth "daughter" Liz,
who makes me laugh.

ACKNOWLEDGMENTS

It has been my pleasure to meet and work with so many people in the preparation of this book: Michael Bentley from Sierra Mountain Minerals, Inc. (a man of high principles), Henry and Carol Kriegel of Kriegel Marketing Group (dedicated and smart), and Rudy Shur from Square One Publishers (Rudy, I've wanted to work with you for a long time).

1

INTRODUCTION
THE BODY ON FIRE

For people suffering from chronic pain, it wasn't good news. And it came right before Christmas, too. First, Vioxx (rofecoxib) was removed from the market on September 30, 2004, because of increased risk of heart attack and stroke. Then on December 17, *USA Today* released a report stating that the over-the-counter pain reliever Aleve (naproxen) had been linked to a 50-percent increased risk of heart attack and stroke. This was followed in rapid succession by similar news about Celebrex (celecoxib).

Studies show that long-term users of both Vioxx and Celebrex have more than twice the risk of heart attacks than those taking a placebo drug. As of this writing, Bextra (valdecoxib) is on the ropes, too, and question marks hang over the entire class of COX-2 inhibitors, part of the family of NSAIDs (nonsteroidal anti-inflammatory drugs). What are people in pain supposed to do?

A GROWING PROBLEM

The anti-inflammatory drugs were introduced into the marketplace for a good reason: increased inflammation. Arthritis—both rheumatoid and osteoarthritis—

has, of course, been around for a long time, as have the other disorders associated with chronic inflammation. (See the inset at right.) Chronic pain is difficult to bear, and people whose joints are painfully swollen are desperate for answers.

The market for effective pain relief is huge and growing. The population of the United States is rapidly aging, and we tend to become more vulnerable to inflammation as we age. Statistics on the number of people who suffer from arthritis vary, but according to the National Institute of Arthritis and Musculoskeletal and Skin Diseases (National Institutes of Health), more than 20 million people may suffer from arthritis. And joint pain is only one type of pain. Inflammation can arise and cause pain in virtually any tissue of the body, except for the brain, where there are few pain receptor sites. But many diseases and disorders of the brain— such as Alzheimer's disease and autism—have now been positively correlated with inflammation. (See the inset on page 5.) When we tally up the number of health conditions that are causally linked to inflammation and the number of people who suffer from those conditions, we are talking about a vast segment of the population.

At the same time that the need for pain relief is growing, our country is experiencing a trend toward self-care, especially among the baby boomers. Sales of dietary supplements marketed to support joint health were $1.025 billion in 2001, and joint health is one of the fastest growing condition categories in the health foods industry. Over $566 million were spent on over-the-counter pharmaceutical joint health products in

Which Disorders Have Been Linked to Inflammation?

When most of us think of inflammation, we think of arthritis and, perhaps, the aches and pains that come with injury. But a number of serious disorders have been causally linked to inflammation—meaning that inflammation is believed to be at the heart of the disease. These disorders include the following:

- ❑ Alzheimer's disease

- ❑ Cardiovascular disease

- ❑ Chronic Obstructive Pulmonary Disease (COPD)

- ❑ Depression

- ❑ Fibromyalgia

- ❑ Inflammatory bowel disease (Crohn's disease and ulcerative colitis)

- ❑ Metabolic syndrome

- ❑ Obesity

- ❑ Osteoarthritis

- ❑ Osteoporosis

- ❑ Rheumatoid arthritis

- ❑ Schizophrenia

2001. Moreover, people are also seeking the counsel of their physicians. Sales of prescription products for joint health totaled $8.114 billion in 2001—an increase of 39 percent over the previous year.

Most of us do not like to take the drugs. When Dr. Jones pulls out his pad and scribbles a prescription to take care of our latest medical problem, we sigh and ask, "Is it really necessary?" Yet, the physician would not prescribe it if he didn't feel it was necessary.

The dilemma is that inflammation is a serious problem. The three top killers in Western society are heart disease, cancer, and diabetes. As stated in the inset on page 3, inflammation is a causative factor in cardiovascular disease, including stroke. Since metabolic syndrome—a collection of symptoms including abdominal and upper-body fat, increased serum cholesterol with an unhealthy imbalance between HDL and LDL cholesterol, and elevated triglycerides—is a precursor of diabetes, we can logically conclude that inflammation may very well be linked with the onset or progression of diabetes. And researchers believe that chronic inflammation may also be a factor in certain forms of cancer. In fact, the research project that recently illuminated the connection between the use of Vioxx and an increased risk of heart disease was seeking to determine just how, and how much, cancer may be causally linked with inflammation.

We hear more and more about rising health-care costs. How much does inflammation contribute to the health-care burden? In a few short years, Medicare will be unable to keep up with the growing costs. Insurance rates are rising faster than the Cost of Living Index, and there is no end in sight to skyrocketing prices. Millions of Americans can no longer even afford health insurance; they surely cannot afford to be ill. If we do not make radical changes in our personal diets and lifestyle, health-care costs may drive this affluent country into bankruptcy. We simply must do something.

THE PROMISE OF THIS BOOK

Fortunately, there is also a lot of good news. According to the United States government, we can completely avoid 80 percent of all health problems if we just make prudent lifestyle and dietary changes. In other words, we can take charge of our health simply by making the right decisions. This is certainly true of inflammation. We don't have to suffer. We don't have to choose between pain and heart disease.

Inflammatory Diseases of the Brain

According to Parris Kidd, PhD, cell biologist and health educator, inflammation plays a major role in many disorders of the brain, but because the brain lacks pain receptors, the afflicted individual is unaware of the inflammation. Among the many inflammatory diseases of the brain, Dr. Kidd lists Parkinson's disease, in which inflammation burns away certain brain zones; multiple sclerosis, which is characterized by on-and-off inflammation; Alzheimer's disease, which involves several processes, including that of inflammation; stroke, which he terms "runaway inflammation"; and autism, in which inflammation is manifested more subtly.

We can lower our risks for developing chronic inflammation—and, at the same time, for developing other life-threatening diseases. We can make the choice to be well.

You are holding in your hands the first proactive step toward wellness—this book. The first step toward getting and staying well is solid information, based on good science and good clinical work. In our media-driven culture, we are bombarded with messages that conflict and confuse. But there is no need to be confused. Good health is really simple, but it has to start with honest, accurate information. I promise to provide science- and common sense-based information in this book, and I promise to make it both interesting and practical.

Step two involves taking a trip to your grocery store. The cornerstone of good health is a healthy diet. A healthy diet is not faddish or quirky. It does not deprive you of basic food groups or sensory pleasure. A healthy diet is simply prepared and frankly delicious! It does, however, require turning your back on most of the American food culture. If you have stopped cooking, you will need to start again, but you are ready to do that anyway, aren't you? You are ready for vibrant health!

Step three toward wellness is restoring balance to your out-of-balance lifestyle. Stress and mental attitudes are directly linked to increased inflammation. I will recommend several changes that you will want to make in the way you live your life, and help you put these suggestions into practice.

Step four towards wellness is a dietary supplement program, using products that have been shown—in both scientific studies and traditional usage—to reduce inflammation and heal tissues. I will provide journal citations so that together, you and your doctor can make an informed decision about the products that will work best for you.

Are you tired of your pain? Are you ready to take charge of your health and get well? Then turn the page and get started . . .

Common Questions and Answers About Natural Remedies

1. Are natural remedies as effective as pharmaceuticals?

Drugs work differently from natural remedies. Pharmaceuticals are generally unnatural substances that impose a greater-than-normal effect on the body, for good and bad. Natural remedies such as vitamins and minerals provide fundamental elements that the body requires for structure and function. When we use nutrients as therapeutic tools, we are generally seeking to restore balance to a body that may, for genetic or other reasons, need one or more nutrients to regain health.

Although drugs may work faster, nutrients and herbal medicines are extremely effective in restoring the body's normal balance. The use of pharmaceuticals always appears hand-in-hand with unwanted effects—side effects. But when natural medicines are used appropriately and wisely, they seldom confer unwanted effects, and often impart other benefits since they work on a deeper (cellular or molecular) level.

While the use of pharmaceutical agents is sometimes necessary and appropriate, you should begin the treatment of any disease condition by restoring a normal nutritional state and normal physiology, which may reduce dependence on drug therapies. This is why it's wise to seek the counsel of a holistic physician when medical treatment is needed.

2. I do not wish to make dietary changes. Will I still benefit from natural remedies?

Yes, but if your diet is full of pro-inflammatory foods like red meat and sugar, it may take longer for you to feel better. Moreover, you may not get the dramatic benefits that can be achieved when natural remedies are paired with a healthful diet.

3. Will I have to take natural anti-inflammatories forever?

Because there are so many causes of chronic inflammation, people react differently to treatment. I suggest that you put the suggested dietary and lifestyle changes in place, and select the natural anti-inflammatory you wish to use. Follow this protocol for a few weeks after the inflammation is relieved and your symptoms are gone. Then reduce use of the anti-inflammatory gradually and keep track of how you feel. If your symptoms do not reappear, you may be able to discontinue using the anti-inflammatory, but if your symptoms return, you will want to resume the protocol.

2

A LITTLE FIRE
IS A GOOD THING

In Chapter 1, you learned that inflammation is a serious and growing problem in Western society. Despite this fact, it is important to understand that our bodies need inflammation. Without inflammation, we would rapidly succumb to invading pathogens that would literally eat us alive.

Only in the past twenty years or so have scientists really begun to understand how the inflammatory process works. We could not comprehend this powerful system until the electron microscope was invented. Then, for the first time in history, we could actually see the amazing battlefield drama unfolding inside us.

A DELICATE BALANCE

The immune system has much to defend against. We are awash in a sea of bacteria—some benign; some pathogenic. We inhale bacteria. We eat microorganisms in our food. We touch our eyes, nose, and mouth, and access is granted. We cut ourselves, and the rupture in our protective skin layer allows bacteria to enter our bloodstream.

We are also bathed in fungi, molds, and yeasts. Some of these primordial life forms are good. They ferment our yogurt, cheese, and wine; allow our bread to rise; and sour our sauerkraut. But they also rupture the delicate membranes lining our respiratory tract and send us into spasms of sneezing and itching eyes. They slaughter the friendly bacteria and cause the burning pain of urinary tract infections.

Some yeasts, like *Candida albicans*, live in balance with bacteria in the colon and vaginal area. But when antibiotics wage a deadly war on bacteria, candida and other yeasts are allowed to proliferate freely. They grow wild, sending tentacles directly through the mucosal barrier into the small and large intestines. As the tentacles of the yeast penetrate the intestinal lining, they create tiny holes through which not only yeasts, but also bacteria can slip directly into the bloodstream. They are not supposed to be there; they are supposed to be confined to the intestinal tract. But as the bacteria invade the bloodstream, the immune system recognizes them as foreign invaders and sets off an immediate alarm. The immune system then engages in a war that continues as long as the breach in the intestinal tract remains open and pathogens continue to enter.

Our environment is hostile. No wonder we so easily succumb to the enemy.

HOW INFLAMMATION WORKS— A BRIEF VISIT TO THE WAR ROOM

Inflammation, a nonspecific internal system of defense, is a fascinating function of the immune system, and is triggered by an injury. The injury can be inflicted by microbes, as in a bacterial invasion; by physical

What Is Arthritis?

When most people hear the word "inflammation," the pain of arthritis comes to mind. In fact, the word arthritis literally means "joint inflammation." But what exactly is arthritis?

Arthritis is not a single disorder, but presents itself in more than one hundred forms and related conditions, including gout, bursitis, carpal tunnel syndrome, celiac disease, fibromyalgia, and lupus. The most common types of this disorder are osteoarthritis and rheumatoid arthritis.

Osteoarthritis (OA) is a disease that causes the breakdown of joint tissue, leading to joint pain and stiffness. Sometimes referred to as "wear and tear" arthritis, osteoarthritis causes bone to rub against bone as the cushioning protection of the tissue is eroded. Although this disease can affect any joint, it most commonly occurs in the hips, knees, feet, and spine, and can also affect some finger joints. OA is one of the oldest and most common diseases in humans, and affects an estimated 21 million adults in the United States.

Rheumatoid arthritis (RA) is a chronic autoimmune disorder, in which an overactive immune system itself destroys the synovium (joint lining), leading to pain, chronic inflammation, tenderness, stiffness, and—eventually—the destruction of the joint. This disorder primarily affects the hands, wrists, elbows, toes, and knees. One of the most disabling form of arthritis, RA is thought to affect more than 6.5 million people in the United States alone.

agents, such as a knife that cuts through the skin; or by chemical agents, such as toxic materials.

There are generally four symptoms that alert us to the inflammatory process: redness, pain, heat, and swelling. Loss of function can also occur, depending on the site of the difficulty. The purpose of the immune response in inflammation is to remove the microbes, toxins, or other foreign material at the site of the injury; prevent the problem from spreading to other organs; and assist in tissue repair. Most of the body's defense elements are located in the blood, and inflammation is the means by which the body's defense cells and chemicals leave the blood and enter the tissue around the injured or infected site.

Inflammation is carried out in three basic stages: the dilation and increased permeability of blood vessels, the influx of immune bodies to the site of the injury, and repair of the damaged tissues.

Immediately after an injury, the blood vessels at the site of the injury expand in diameter and become increasing permeable to give more immune bodies, such as antibodies, access to the site. The increased blood flow also allows repair materials, such as blood-clotting substances, to enter the area, and assists in "garbage removal," including the removal of invading microorganisms and dead cells.

The immune response is rapid. Within minutes after the injury, you can see the telltale signs of inflammation—the heat, redness, and swelling—that occur as a result of the increased blood flow. As the heat increases, the speed of metabolic reactions increases as well, making the immune response proceed more rapidly.

At the same time swelling and pain occur, tissue damage resulting from the injury causes *fibrinogen*— the blood-clotting factor synthesized by the liver—to rush to the scene. There, fibrinogen converts into a thick network of fibrin threads, or blood clots, that localize the infection, stop the bleeding, and attract phagocytes—specialized cells that are developed in the bone marrow.

Phagocytes—which include the immune cells known as *neutrophils* and *macrophages*—constitute the body's first line of defense against infectious agents and other substances that penetrate the body's physical barriers. In a process called *phagocytosis*, the phagocytes engulf and absorb invading microbes, as well as waste materials and other foreign bodies. After the phagocytes have eaten to satiation, they die and become one of the constituents of pus, which also contains decomposing body tissue and bacteria or other microorganisms. Eventually, the pus is absorbed by the body. The body then goes about repairing the damaged area, and all signs of inflammation disappear.

Our brief description of the inflammatory process wouldn't be complete without a look at a few of the many substances that enable this immune response to occur. Inflammation couldn't take place without the action of tissue hormones called *histamines* and blood proteins known as *kinins*, which cause increased blood flow, enhanced permeability of capillaries, and pain. *Leukotrienes* and *prostaglandins*, which are synthesized throughout the body, also help activate the inflammatory process, causing swelling and pain. Many other substances also take part in the complex response known as inflammation. While all of these substances are vital to the defense of the body, as you can see, they also are primarily responsible for the discomfort associated with the inflammatory process.

When it works appropriately, inflammation is a magnificent response designed to protect and heal the body. Inflammation can actually prevent us from dying of injury or infection. A problem occurs, however, when this response becomes chronic. It can then flare out of control, creating pain and damage throughout the system.

FUELING THE FIRE

Chapter 2 described the lifesaving actions of a healthy immune system. You now understand that inflammation is an important process that, when it occurs appropriately, enables the body to protect itself from immune challenges and heal itself from injury.

But, as you learned in the first chapter of this book, inflammation can be deadly. When the fires of chronic inflammation continually rage on and on, they can literally consume the body. There is a huge difference between an acute inflammation that competently responds to a short-lived assault and then subsides, and a chronic inflammation that burns for years, tearing down the host.

An appropriate acute inflammatory process may occur when you cut your skin, when you eat spoiled foods, or when you are exposed to an overload of pollen during hay fever season. Your body is equipped to handle that type of exposure; it is what your immune system was designed to do.

An inappropriate chronic inflammatory process occurs when the assault is no longer confined to a discrete area, such as the site of a wound, or a discrete period of time, such as hay fever season. When exposure to an offending substance is prolonged or when the immune system becomes so compromised that it can no longer respond appropriately, inflammation can flare out of control and become chronic.

Why has chronic inflammation become a growing problem in our society? What is fueling the fire? The answer appears to lie in our society itself—in the way we eat and the way we live our lives.

OUR INFLAMMATORY DIET

A developing body of scientific investigation and clinical study shows that modern dietary and lifestyle factors appear to increase our risk of developing chronic inflammation. And the factor most responsible for this increased risk is the Western food culture.

If we had lived prior to the dawn of the twentieth century, our eating habits would have been drastically different from what they are today. Our ancestors ate from the earth. They pulled fish from the streams and oceans, and hunted for wild game. They churned warm cream into butter or pressed the oil out of olives and seeds. They coaxed eggs from under mother hens as they nested in the fields.

Our ancestors snipped bitter and sweet greens from fields and gardens. They plucked fruits and vegetables—fully ripe and bursting with nutrition—from trees, bushes, and vines. The produce was organic. Farmers tilled decaying plant material back into the soil so it could give life to new crops. They irrigated their fields with local waters that were rich in minerals.

Prior to the twentieth century, people ate seasonally when food was at its peak. And they ate locally; nothing was picked green and shipped long distances in refrigerated trucks. Their food nearly pulsated with

life. They rarely suffered from "diseases of civiliza-
tion" like heart disease and arthritis.

Now, we eat from plastic boxes and cardboard
containers. We ingest pseudo-foods designed in a
chemist's laboratory, or foods that have been geneti-
cally modified to resemble something else. We slurp
sugary chemical brews. We fry our food in oils that
have been degraded into toxins.

Of course, most of us know that pseudo-foods are
not healthy. But the fact is that even those of us who
strive to eat a healthful diet may unwittingly be choosing foods that either create or worsen inflammatory
conditions. Some of the most inflammatory foods, for
instance, include beef, wheat, corn, potatoes, eggplants, and tomatoes. How do these foods—as well as
"fake" foods like sugary sodas and processed oils—
lead to chronic inflammation? Let's find out.

Beef and Pork

Both beef and pork have a strong inflammatory effect
on the body. There are several reasons these meats "set
the body on fire."

First, farm-raised beef and pork are rich sources
of *arachidonic acid*, a type of fatty acid that metabolizes
into specific hormones such as prostaglandins and
leukotrienes—substances that you read about in Chapter 2 because they play a major role in the inflammatory process.

It is important to understand that prostaglandins
are subdivided into three groups: the prostaglandin 1
(PGE1), prostaglandin 2 (PGE2), and prostaglandin 3
(PGE3) series. PGE1 and PGE3 are actually anti-

inflammatory substances that reduce inflammation, lower blood pressure, help regulate heartbeat, and have other beneficial effects on the body. These anti-inflammatory prostaglandins are constructed from omega-3 fatty acids, which are derived from fish and plant sources.

PGE2, however, is a pro-inflammatory prostaglandin, constructed from the arachidonic acid found in farm-raised beef and pork. Animals that are raised in the wild are able to produce a higher concentration of omega-3 fatty acids and a lower concentration of arachidonic acid, but it is difficult to find wild-raised animals in today's marketplace. The result is that our intake of essential fatty acids tilts toward the inflammatory fats.

The second cause of meat's inflammatory effects has to do with the body's pH. Different tissues of the body each function best at a specific pH. One of the most important measures of a healthy body pH is that of the blood, which must be slightly alkaline—somewhere between 7.35 and 7.45—to maintain optimum health. It is dangerous for blood pH to fluctuate beyond those ranges, either lower toward acidity or higher toward alkalinity. And when the blood becomes too acidic—a condition that is far more common than over-alkalinity—inflammation is likely to result.

What does this have to do with meat? Beef and pork, as well as other animal proteins, skew the important acid-alkaline balance toward inflammatory acidity because they leave an acidic residue after digestion. According to one peer review journal article, acidosis (over-acidity) has been observed in cases of chronic joint inflammation and tumors. Over-acidity has also been found to contribute to pain by stimulating the hormonal messenger Substance P, which is known to enhance pain levels.[1]

Grains

Most people are aware of the United States Department of Agriculture Food Guide Pyramid, which recommends six to eleven servings a day of grains in the form of bread, cereal, rice, and pasta. While grains—and especially whole grains—contain valuable nutrients, many of them have been found to have certain negative effects on the body.

First, it should be noted that for a good segment of the population, grains have proven to be fattening. This, alone, is a problem for many well-known reasons. However, what most people do not know is that obesity has been linked to inflammation. Moreover, grains are for the most part acidifying. Just like meat, grains leave an acidic ash upon digestion, thus lowering the pH of the body and contributing to inflammation. Finally, wheat and other gluten-containing grains are one of the top three food allergens. Some grains may, therefore, also contribute to inflammation through the allergy response.

Because grains are such a rich source of nutrients, I am not recommending that you remove them totally from your diet. However, I do recommend that you eat only modest amounts of those grains that have been shown to contribute least to inflammation. The "good" grains include millet, quinoa, rice (especially brown rice), spelt, kamut, and amaranth. I also suggest that, whenever possible, you eat whole grains, as they have been found less problematic than refined grains.

Other Acidifying Foods

Unfortunately, beef, pork, and grains are not the only foods that have an acidifying effect on the body. Other foods with the same effect include sugar and high-sugar products; carbonated beverages; alcoholic beverages; and all caffeine products, including chocolate, cocoa, tea, and all forms of coffee, including decaffeinated coffee. Because the regular consumption of any of these foods compromises the ability of the body to maintain a healthy pH, they all can contribute to inflammation.

Another food that can adversely affect pH is processed vegetable oil. In addition, these oils deplete the body of anti-inflammatory omega-3 fatty acids, and encourage the synthesis of PGE2, the pro-inflammatory prostaglandin.

Foods in the Nightshade Family

The nightshade family of plants comprises about 2,600 species worldwide, including herbs, shrubs, trees, vines, and major food crops such as potatoes, tomatoes, eggplants, and chile peppers. Also included in this group is the tobacco plant. Some of the plants in this family—deadly nightshade, for instance—are known to be poisonous. Others, as you know, constitute an important part of many peoples' diets. Unfortunately, even these seemingly benign plants can often cause problems.

All vegetables in the nightshade family contain a

chemical alkaloid that is an irritant, and can contribute to inflammation. People who suffer from arthritis, for instance, sometimes find that pain and swelling increase after they eat vegetables from this family of plants. The irritating alkaloids have been found in greatest amounts in the green spots found on improperly stored potatoes, and in green tomatoes. The bitter taste of these vegetables is a telltale sign of the presence of alkaloids.

According to holistic physician Dr. Jonathan Wright, laboratory tests cannot be used to determine if an individual has a sensitivity to foods in the nightshade family. If you suffer from inflammation and want to discover if these foods are worsening your condition, the best course of action is to eliminate the nightshade vegetables from your diet for at least one month and possibly more, because it sometimes takes over three months for symptoms to subside. Note any improvements brought about by the removal of the foods. Then reintroduce them one by one, carefully observing any changes so that you can pinpoint which vegetables, if any, are contributing to your condition.

Oxalate-Rich Foods

You have just learned about several groups of foods that are known to create inflammatory conditions in the body. In many people, elimination of one or more of these groups can help bring the symptoms of inflammation under control. But when these dietary modifications do not have the desired result, another group of foods should be considered.

It is been found that some people who suffer from

extreme pain, particularly in the vulvar (vaginal) region or in the urinary tract, are victims of oxalate-rich foods. Oxalates are colorless crystalline organic acids commonly found in plant foods such as spinach, beets, wheat bran, peanuts, chocolate, and tea. Biomedical research consultant Dr. Clive Solomon studies oxalates in relationship to vulvar and other pain. According to his work, vulvar pain is a connective tissue disorder that is worsened by high-oxalate foods, which causes tissue to collapse and thin, "making the nerves more accessible to pain-producing molecules." This results in a chronic inflammatory state. People with this condition often describe the pain as "being filled with crushed glass." That description is not surprising since the oxalate crystals look like shards of glass.

The body produces its own oxalates in the liver and other tissues. Microbes can manufacture oxalates in the intestines, and of course, we consume oxalates in some commonly eaten foods. In the body, oxalates chemically bond to minerals such as sodium, potassium, magnesium, and calcium, creating oxalate salts. These salts can form in the kidneys and/or urinary tract, in the vulvar region, and elsewhere, leading to kidney stone formation, vulvar pain, and, it is thought, pain in other areas of the body.

According to the Vulvar Pain Foundation, the inflammation caused by oxalate-rich foods is best treated by avoiding these foods, while supplementing with calcium citrate and an amino sugar called N-Acetyl Glucosamine (NAG). Foods that are rich in oxalates include apples, apricots, beets, blackberries, blueberries, broccoli, Brussels sprouts, carrots, celery, chard, chives, cocoa and cocoa-containing products, collard greens, Concord grapes, cranberries and cranberry juice, currants, dandelion greens, endives, gooseberries, green beans, kale, leeks, okra, oranges, parsnips, peanuts, pecans, raspberries, rhubarb, soy products such as soy milk and tofu, spinach, strawberries, sweet potatoes, tea, turnip greens, wheat germ, and white potatoes. As in the case of the nightshade vegetables discussed previously, only an elimination diet, followed by the systematic reintroduction of foods, can help you determine if high-oxalate foods are causing a problem.

OUR INFLAMMATORY LIFESTYLE

Although you may have never thought about it before, our language correlates emotional stress with inflam-

---

Creating a Low-Oxalate Diet

As you can see from the list of oxalate-rich foods found on pages 22 and 23, the fruits, vegetables, and other products that can contribute to inflammation through the formation of oxalate salt are many. How, then, do you create a low-oxalate diet? The Vulvar Pain Foundation—a nonprofit organization devoted to research and education—has compiled lists of "Can Eat" and "Cannot Eat" foods to help people avoid products that can worsen inflammatory conditions. To receive these lists, simply contact the foundation. (Visit their website at www.vulvarpainfoundation.org.)

mation. "Burning with anger," "I was so angry I saw red," "Fiery temper"—these phrases all show how we link anger and stress with the redness and fire of the inflammatory process. Is this simply a matter of semantics, or is there a real connection between emotional stress and the inflammatory conditions that plague our society?

You may be surprised to learn that our frantically paced lifestyles, fraught with stress, may be setting our bodies on fire. Recent research on inflammatory disease points a guilty finger to stress, anger, unforgiveness, burnout, shame, guilt, fear, sleep deprivation, and loneliness.

The common ground between attitude and inflammation lies in a substance called *C-reactive protein* (CRP), an indicator of inflammation in the arteries. People who are prone to anger, hostility, and depression release more of this powerful substance. And this substance, in turn, leads to narrowing and inflammation of the arteries.

In a recent study published in *Psychosomatic Medicine*, 127 healthy men and women were assessed for anger, hostility, and depression. Researchers then measured their CRP levels. The study found that adults who struggled with depression, anger, or hostility had levels of CRP that were several times higher than those of happier, calmer adults. And the higher the mood disorder, the higher the levels of CRP.

One of the researchers noted that anger, hostility, and depression tend to cluster in the same individual, which increases the risk even further. People who tend to be hostile often react to events with anger, and the resulting emotional storm leads to symptoms of depression.[2]

Anger, hostility, and depression are not the only emotions linked with inflammation. Guilt and loneliness play a role, too, along with fear, burnout, and shame. Think of the expression, "I felt like it was eating me alive." Shame and other emotions may literally "eat us alive" as they nurture inflammation.

Shame has been found to be a more powerful influence on inflammation than guilt. Guilt is often short-term in nature. We realize that we messed up and vow not to repeat our mistake. Shame, however, is more difficult to handle and tends to get bottled up, with no release valve. Researchers have found that this emotion increases the activity of *cytokines*—messengers of the immune system that signal an inflammatory disease process.[3] Shame also appears to be "dose related." Individuals with higher levels of shame also have higher levels of cytokine activity.

Other measures of inflammation have also been shown to correlate with stress. According to one study, clinical depression caused by stress is linked to higher levels of an immune complex called *interleukin-6* (IL-6), a measure of inflammation.[4] In yet another study, which focused on the parents of cancer patients, researchers found that stress lowered the parents' sensitivity to *glucocorticoids*—steroid hormones that are frequently used to treat inflammatory disorders such as arthritis, asthma, and liver inflammation. Stress, it has been found, impairs the immune system's capacity to respond to normal hormonal cues that signal the end of an inflammatory attack after infection or injury.

The body simply doesn't receive the hormonal message to shut the inflammatory process down.

Before we leave the subject of stress, it is important to recognize that emotional stress isn't the only culprit in the stress-inflammation connection. Physical stressors such as illness and hard physical work have also been found to play a role in chronic inflammation.

IT'S ALL AROUND US

It would appear that we're driving the inflammatory process ourselves through both our diet and our lifestyle choices. We're throwing kerosene on the fire,

---

Obesity, Depression, and Inflammation

Everyone knows the deadly effects that obesity can have on the human body. Recent research, however, has shown that obesity is even more dangerous when paired with depression.

According to a study published in *Brain, Behavior and Immunity*, greater depression in obese men resulted in significantly higher levels of C-reactive protein (CRP), the marker of inflammation first discussed on page 24. Interestingly, depression was *not* linked to higher levels of CRP in non-obese men.[5] For many people, then, the relief of inflammation may require a two-pronged approach—both a diet designed to decrease weight and appropriate treatment for emotional stress.

even while we're trying to extinguish it. What is the sense in that? If inflammation is an issue involving the whole body, we need a "whole body approach."

Yet, as we all know, many people avoid making dietary and lifestyle changes, and prefer instead to explore the world of pharmaceuticals. Certainly, the drug industry has created a number of products designed to reduce inflammation. If you're interested in pharmaceutical solutions, you'll want to turn to the next chapter. Later, in Chapter 5, we will explore a holistic approach to inflammatory disease.

4

THE PHARMACEUTICAL APPROACH

The invention of antibiotics signaled the arrival of "medicine by magic." Before antibiotics arrived on the medical scene, patients were at the mercy of bacteria, and indeed, bacterial and other infections were the leading cause of death throughout human history. But when Sir Arthur Fleming discovered penicillin in 1929, and doctors realized that the simple administration of a pill could magically conquer many diseases, a new age of medicine dawned. No longer were doctors trained in herbology and other natural remedies; they went to school to learn how to administer medications. And as the number and types of drugs proliferated, medicine became big business—huge business, in fact.

With the introduction of effective drugs, it became easier to treat illness because physicians did not have to get involved in the messy business of people's lives—how they ate, how they washed their hands, how they handled stress. Pills were dispensed to make all the bad things go away. This is not to discount the tremendous advantages that modern medicine can provide. Personally, I enjoy living in a world where I can get an antibiotic if the need truly arises, and where competent anesthesia is available if I must get a tooth pulled. We need medicine; no question about it. If you are in pain, you need to be relieved of pain, and pharmaceutical companies have invested a great deal of money to learn how pain works and what we can do to shut it down.

Problems arise, however, when the medical disorder is not short-term, but a long-term problem that requires constant medication—medication that can have adverse effects when used in great and continual doses. And, as everyone with arthritis and other inflammatory diseases knows, those little pills don't always offer relief.

What is the pharmaceutical approach to inflammation? Let's take a look.

THE FIRST NSAIDS

In the early 1900s, when Friedrich Bayer & Co. introduced aspirin tablets to the public, it is doubtful that the company knew how successful the drug would be. But it was successful from the very start. Derived from a substance found in the bark of the white willow tree, and then buffered to minimize harm to the stomach, aspirin was embraced as a means of treating headache, relieving the pain of arthritis and other inflammatory ailments, and lowering fever. In fact, aspirin became one of the most successful medicines of all time. It was also the first nonsteroidal anti-inflammatory drug, or NSAID. Although it had been buffered, in many people, aspirin still had the effect of irritating the stomach, and in some people, it even led to the development of ulcers.

Later, other NSAIDs were developed in an effort to provide relief while lessening side effects. The most common anti-inflammatories used today are ibuprofen, sold under trade names such as Advil, Motrin, and Nuprin; and naproxen, which is best known as the drug Aleve. But when these new NSAIDs are used on a continual basis to treat a chronic inflammatory disease such as arthritis, side effects still occur.

To understand both how NSAIDs work and how they create problems, we must go back to earlier discussions of the inflammatory process. Chapter 2 briefly mentioned the role that prostaglandins play in inflammation. Later, in Chapter 3, you learned that there are actually three types of prostaglandins—prostaglandin 1 (PGE1), prostaglandin 2 (PGE2), and prostaglandin 3 (PGE3). PGE1 and PGE3 are actually *anti*-inflammatory substances, and PGE2 is *pro*-inflammatory. All of these prostaglandins are useful. During the inflammatory process, PGE2 allows the body to respond to injury by producing inflammation as part of the immune response. Once the body has dealt with the emergency, PGE1 and PGE3 work to eliminate the inflammation. These anti-inflammatory substances also stimulate the formation of the protective lining of the stomach, normalize platelet function, and enhance the flow of blood to the kidneys.

The NSAIDs aspirin, ibuprofen, and naproxen work by stopping the production of *all* prostaglandins. They do this by interfering with an enzyme called *cyclooxgenase*, or COX, which is necessary for the production of prostaglandins. The problem is that these drugs stop not only the inflammatory process that causes the pain of arthritis and many other disorders, but also the anti-inflammatory process that protects the stomach lining.

When the drugs are taken on a continual basis, the result is often indigestion, nausea, and worse.

COX-2 INHIBITOR NSAIDS

For many years, scientists did not understand how aspirin and other NSAIDs worked. But in the early 1970s, when they first recognized the action of NSAIDs on prostaglandins, they began to explore ways in which safer anti-inflammatory drugs could be developed. For a moment, let's go back to our discussion of the COX enzyme, and learn a little more about it.

Scientists have identified three forms of COX enzymes. The COX-1 enzyme is involved in the production of those prostaglandins that regulate pain, blood clotting, blood flow to the kidneys, and the mucus production that protects the lining of the stomach. This enzyme is found in most body tissues, with levels remaining stable throughout the body.

The COX-2 enzyme is involved in the production of those prostaglandins responsible for inflammation and the pain associated with the inflammatory process. Unlike the COX-1 enzyme, this enzyme is not normally present in the cells. Instead, when a bacterial invasion or other injury occurs, white blood cells stimulate the production of the COX-2 enzyme at the site of the injury.

Finally, the COX-3 enzyme appears to regulate pain and fever. Research into this enzyme is still in its infancy. It is believed, however, that the drug acetaminophen—which can relieve pain and fever, but *cannot* control inflammation—may work by interfering with the action of COX-3.

As scientists explored the different COX enzymes, they saw the advantages of targeting only the COX-2 enzyme—the enzyme responsible for the inflammatory process. And so in 1999, manufacturers introduced a new class of NSAIDs called *COX-2 inhibitors*, which selectively inhibit the pro-inflammatory COX-2 enzyme while having minimal or no effects on the stomach-protecting COX-1 enzyme.

The COX-2 inhibitors were greeted with enthusiasm as first Celebrex (celecoxib), then Vioxx (rofecoxib), and then Bextra (valdecoxib) entered the market. Unlike the traditional NSAIDs, which came in over-the-counter strengths, these were all prescription drugs. Yet despite the fact that they required a prescription and cost far more than the traditional NSAIDs, the COX-2 inhibitors contributed to a dramatic increase in NSAID use. Arthritis sufferers were eager to try medications that could ease joint pain and inflammation without causing gastrointestinal upset and other side effects associated with earlier NSAIDs.

But as most people know, while COX-2 inhibitors may not pose a threat to the stomach, they are not without side effects. As early as 1999, the National Academy of Science warned that COX-2 inhibitors increase the risk of stroke, heart attack, and blood-clotting disorders. Then in 2001, cardiologists at the Cleveland Clinic analyzed clinical trials of COX-2 inhibitors to determine if these drugs have any effect on cardiovascular health. In a trial involving 8,059 people given either Vioxx or the NSAID diclofenac, patients taking the COX-2 drug were found twice as likely to suffer a cardiovascular event such as heart attack or stroke.

Among those subjects who had a history of heart disease, the risk of a cardiovascular event was found to be *four* times greater when using Vioxx rather than a traditional NSAID. In September 2004, Merck and Co., the manufacturer of Vioxx, removed the drug from the market. According to numerous reports, upwards of 140,000 people may have suffered a heart event as a consequence of taking either Vioxx or one of the other COX-2 inhibitors.

It should be noted that no one knows exactly why the new class of NSAIDs appears to increase the risk of heart disease. One theory that has been offered, however, is that these drugs suppress the body's production of prostacyclin, a prostaglandin that dilates the blood vessels and inhibits the formation of blood clots.

THE SMOLDERING FIRES OF INFLAMMATION

Before we leave the subject of NSAIDs—both traditional forms and COX-2 inhibitors—it's worthwhile to look at them from another point of view. Anti-inflammatory medications do serve a purpose, and studies show that for many people, they may be perfectly safe when taken in low doses for a restricted period of time. But doctors point out that neither these drugs nor any other drugs cure arthritis. They damp the fires of inflammation, temporarily relieving the pain of arthritis and other inflammatory disorders, but the fire still smolders. Meanwhile, chronic inflammation continues to destroy synovial tissue, erode bone structure, and perhaps set the stage for cardiovascular disease. In the case of long-term inflammation, a better solution—a holistic solution—seems to be in order.

A HOLISTIC APPROACH

Earlier, in Chapter 3, you saw that the foods we eat and the way we live our lives is fueling the fire of inflammatory disease. In fact, the American food culture is, for the most part, an inflammation-promoting diet, with a heavy emphasis on pro-inflammatory sugar, soft drinks, alcoholic beverages, beef, and grains. And our high-stress lives further exacerbate the problem.

You can unquestionably derive great benefits from natural anti-inflammatories—products you'll be learning about in Chapter 6. But trying to solve the problem of inflammation without addressing the core issues of diet and lifestyle is like pouring kerosene on a fire even as you are trying to extinguish it. That's why this chapter takes a *holistic approach* to the problem of inflammation, meaning that it focuses not only on relieving any existing inflammatory condition, but also on using dietary and lifestyle changes to prevent illness in the future and maintain radiant good health.

DESIGNING AN ANTI-INFLAMMATORY DIET

Chapter 3 discussed the major pro-inflammatory foods: beef and pork; certain grains; and various other common products, including sugar, soft drinks, alcohol, chocolate, tea, coffee, and processed vegetable oils. In addition, for some people, certain other foods can cause or worsen inflammatory conditions. If you have not already read that chapter, it would be worth your while to take the few minutes needed to "digest" it. It's important to understand not only *what* should be avoided, but also *why* it should be avoided.

Goodbye, Morning Coffee

When I was a young adult, we drank plain old coffee, perhaps with a little milk and sugar. Now we drink giant lattes, cappuccinos, frappuccinos, and dozens of other gourmet drinks, all with pro-inflammatory coffee as the base, as well as far more than a splash of inflammatory (and fattening) milk. We all know that too much coffee makes it difficult for some people to sleep. But can this common beverage be truly harmful?

In a study of 1,514 men and 1,528 women with a mean age of forty-five years, it was found that compared with people who don't drink coffee, men who consumed more than 200 milliliters of coffee per day had 30-percent higher levels of C-reactive protein and greater concentrations of other markers of inflammation. And women who consumed more than 200 milliliters of coffee per day had even higher levels of inflammatory markers.[1] While 200 milliliters may sound like a lot, keep in mind that it is a little less than 7 ounces—not even a full cup! The lesson to be learned? If you're trying to reduce inflammation, say good-bye to your morning cup of coffee and hello to an anti-inflammatory cup of green tea.

Now that you know what you shouldn't eat, let's focus on a more pleasant topic—all the foods you can and should eat not only to relieve pain and inflammation, but also to promote overall good health. Are you ready to be well? Are you ready to make changes to insure the health of your bones, joints, and muscles? Are you willing to forego the pleasures of a few familiar foods in order to heal your body?

If so, you will now begin a marvelous journey toward health—an adventure that begins in your kitchen. Let's start the journey by looking at the food groups that are primarily *anti*-inflammatory:

❑ Fruits.

❑ Vegetables.

❑ Seafood—especially omega-3-rich fish such as salmon, sardines, mackerel, and mullet.

❑ Cold-pressed olive and macadamia nut oils.

❑ Raw nuts, particularly almonds and walnuts.

❑ Lamb, veal, and poultry (organic or wild raised when possible).

❑ Water.

❑ Green tea.

What makes the above foods fit into the anti-inflammatory category?

First and foremost, the above foods are alkalizing, meaning that when they are digested and metabolized, they produce an alkaline ash in the body. As you learned in Chapter 3, acidifying foods promote inflammation. Alkalizing foods, on the other hand, *lower* the potential for inflammation. Be aware that even citrus fruits, which are acidic, leave an *alkaline* ash when they are digested, and therefore have an alkalizing effect on the body.

Second, the first two foods listed—fruits and vegetables—are good sources of important minerals. Because minerals are alkaline, the body overcomes the effects of an acidic diet by using certain minerals as buffering agents. If adequate amounts of these minerals are not available in the diet, the body pulls them out of bones and teeth—a situation that can lead to osteoporosis and a variety of other disorders.

Finally, fruits and vegetables are a rich source of antioxidant nutrients, which have been shown to protect against coronary disease, cancer, and other serious disorders. For all of these reasons, I recommend that you incorporate at least seven servings of vegetables and two servings of fruit into your daily diet. Choose fresh over canned and frozen, and whenever possible, select produce that is organic and freshly harvested. Fruits and vegetables are, in fact, the cornerstone of the anti-inflammatory diet.

Of course, we cannot live on fruits and vegetables alone. Balance is the key to a healthy anti-inflammatory diet. Seafood and other animal proteins provide us with the building blocks we need to keep our bodies strong. And certain fish, of course, are high in the anti-inflammatory omega-3 fatty acids. Both olive and macadamia nut oils have been included because they, too, provide important fatty acids. Nuts are a treasure-trove of nutrients, including essential fatty acids.

Green tea has been found to have anti-inflammatory properties, and to provide a range of important antioxidants. And, as we all know, we each need at least eight glasses of water a day to prevent dehydration and to keep our bodies functioning optimally.

Now you know what foods should be avoided and what foods have anti-inflammatory benefits. But you may not be sure how to use these do's and don'ts to construct a sound diet. The sample menus found on page 41 should prove helpful. Note that they are *sample* menus, and are only intended to serve as examples of the anti-inflammatory meals you can eat over a four-day period. Use them as a springboard for

---

Now There's Proof!

For many years, we've all heard that a diet high in whole fruits and vegetables, legumes, fish, and poultry is healthy—better for our hearts, and better for our bodies overall. But is there proof that people who maximize their intake of these foods actually have a lower incidence of inflammatory disease?

In a study of 732 women between the ages of forty-three and sixty-nine years of age, researchers found that higher intakes of fruits, vegetables, legumes, fish, and poultry were associated with lower levels of C-reactive protein (CRP)—an indication of inflammation. On the other hand, diets characterized by higher intakes of red and processed meats, sweets, desserts, French fries, and refined grains were associated with several markers of inflammation.[2] Now we know!

creating your own diet—a diet that you can fully enjoy with your family as you reap its anti-inflammatory benefits. Just be sure to keep the following guidelines in mind:

❑ Avoid the most common allergens–wheat, corn, and dairy—as well as any foods that pose a particular problem to you. (We'll discuss that later in the chapter.) To steer clear of gluten, the substance in wheat that causes problems for so many people, look for the words "Gluten-Free" (or "GF") on the baked goods you buy.

❑ Use foods that are as close to nature as possible—fresh organically grown produce, for instance.

❑ Include seven servings of vegetables and two servings of fruits a day. (Note that a serving is about the size of your clenched fist, so a large salad easily provides three or more servings of vegetables.)

❑ Include only modest portions of the following anti-inflammatory grains—millet, quinoa, rice (especially brown rice), spelt, kamut, and amaranth.

❑ Rotate the sources of protein—which, of course, should exclude beef and pork—so that you eat the same protein no more frequently than every four days. This strategy will help prevent the development of new food sensitivities.

All of the recommended recipes in the following menus can be found in the back of this book, beginning on page 86.

SAMPLE ANTI-INFLAMMATORY MENUS

Day One

Breakfast: Northwest Salmon Hash (page 87).

Lunch: Large bowl of Multi-Bean Soup (page 88), rice crackers, fresh fruit of your choice.

Dinner: Salmon Poached in White Wine (page 96), Vegetable Risotto (page 97), crudités (raw vegetables), Roasted Asparagus (page 95).

Snack: Fresh fruit or raw nut mix.

Day Two

Breakfast: Rice-based protein drink blended with fresh fruit and flax seed or olive oil.

Lunch: Curried Chickpeas and Kale (page 91), spelt bread.

Dinner: Braised Lamb (page 92), mashed potatoes, steamed carrots and peas.

Snack: Fresh fruit.

Day Three

Breakfast: 2 poached or fried eggs, 2 slices gluten-free bread (millet is good).

Lunch: Roasted Red Pepper Hummus (page 90) with rice crackers and fresh vegetables.

Dinner: Your favorite rotisserie or roasted chicken, baked sweet potatoes, large salad with several colorful vegetables topped with olive oil and a splash of balsamic vinegar.

Snack: Fresh fruit or raw nut mix.

Day Four

Breakfast: Brown Rice with Fruit and Nuts (page 86).

Lunch: A Salad You Could Enjoy Every Day (page 89).

Dinner: Southeast Asian Seafood Stew (page 94) over quinoa or rice.

Snack: Half avocado with a splash of olive oil and balsamic vinegar.

Once you start eating a diet rich in inflammation-fighting foods, you'll see that it has many benefits, not the least of which is great flavor. Because of all the fruits and vegetables, for instance, this diet is relatively low in calories and will help your weight remain at a healthy level. And the rich supply of nutrients it provides will enable you to fight the many disorders associated with aging. So not only will you feel and look wonderful, but you will enjoy your good health for many years!

While the dietary guidelines presented above will provide great benefits for many people, they may not be sufficient for every individual who suffers from inflammatory conditions. As you learned in Chapter 3, some foods cause problems only for certain people. How can you identify the specific foods that may be creating or worsening your own health problems? Let's see.

DEALING WITH FOOD ALLERGIES AND SENSITIVITIES

Earlier in the book, I mentioned how allergies are pro-inflammatory. But allergies are just one type of reac-

---

The Mediterranean Diet

In recent years, nearly everyone has heard about the health benefits of the Mediterranean diet—a diet high in fruits and vegetables, beans, nuts, seeds, olive oil, fish, and poultry, and low in dairy products and red meat. Most literature has emphasized the heart-healthy effects of the diet. Is it also helpful in the battle against inflammation?

Studies have shown that those who adhere to a Mediterranean diet do indeed show a significant (20-percent) reduction in levels of C-reactive protein, an important marker for inflammation. This diet has also been found to significantly lower levels of other inflammatory markers, including interleukin-6 (17 percent lower), tumor necrosis factor-alpha (16 percent lower), fibrinogen (6 percent lower), homocysteine (15 percent lower), and white blood cells (14 percent lower). It's wonderful to know that a diet that's so delicious is also beneficial to the body in so many ways.[3]

---

tion that can cause inflammation. Food intolerances of all kinds can create this condition. What's the difference between an allergy and a food intolerance? A *food intolerance* is a condition in which a particular adverse reaction occurs after eating a particular food or food ingredient. A *food allergy* is actually a type of food intolerance, and can be defined as a condition in which a specific *immune reaction* occurs in response to consuming a particular food, causing histamine to be released. All allergies are intolerances, but not all intolerances are allergies.

Food intolerances, including allergies, affect a large number of people, many of whom have never been diagnosed because it is often difficult to associate commonly eaten foods with symptoms. In some cases, a reaction may occur directly after eating a food. Someone who is allergic to artichokes, for instance, may find her throat growing itchy and closing up soon after she's taken her first bite of the offending food. But in some cases, a reaction may not take place for hours or even days after consumption. And since so many of the dishes we eat contain a number of different foods, we may not associate our reaction with the substance that actually caused it.

Intolerances can affect any part of the body with any type of symptom. I have known people to be allergic to bananas, shrimp, corn chips, almonds, sesame seeds, and more. And I have seen them react with headaches, burning and itching eyes, ADD/ADHD, bouts of diarrhea, constipation, nausea, abdominal pain, joint pain, severe muscle pain, severe back pain, depression, and symptoms of autism or Pervasive Developmental Disorder (PDD). The list goes on and on because the body is very creative in expressing unhappiness with dietary choices.

I am personally reactive to garlic, chicken, eggs, corn, and all grains except rice. My list of problem foods covers many that are generally regarded as being healthy. As it has been said, "One man's food is another man's poison." Although I do not notice the flicker of inflammatory pain after eating just a little garlic, if I eat a larger amount two or three days in a row, a raging inferno cripples me. I literally cannot walk.

While any food can trigger an allergic response, the most common culprits are wheat, corn, and dairy, followed by soy, shellfish, citrus, chocolate, nuts, and so on. Wheat, corn, and dairy are well known for causing mild to severe gastrointestinal inflammation, mental and emotional disorders, and all types of muscular and joint pain. As discussed in Chapter 3, some people are also highly sensitive to nightshade vegetables such as tomatoes and potatoes. People who experience inflammatory symptoms as a result of eating these foods on a regular basis probably do not associate the food with the pain—until they completely eliminate the offending foods for a period of time, feel better, and

---

Important Allergy Testing

Standard allergy testing is not completely reliable, and often detects only immediate reactions to about 100 dietary and environmental substances. Clearly, the person who suffers from delayed reactions would not be helped by these tests. But a better test is available.

The ELISA/ACT LRA is a combination of the Enzyme-Linked Immunosorbant Assay (ELISA), the Advanced Cell Test (ACT), and the Lymphocyte Response Assay (LRA). This simple blood test can detect the body's delayed immune response to as many as 400 substances. Developed by ELISA/ACT Biotechnologies, the test must be prescribed by your physician.

reintroduce the foods to their diets. Their discomfort then is often quite extreme—an exaggerated response to the offending substance.

If you are suffering from inflammation and you suspect that certain foods are causing a problem, I suggest that you eliminate them from your diet for at least three months. Do you feel better? Are you experiencing less pain and stiffness? Better flexibility and mobility? If so, it is likely that food intolerances are stoking the fires of your inflammation.

Once your symptoms have disappeared, you may try to reintroduce the foods one by one, noting your reaction so that you can pinpoint the offending substance. But be careful. If you are truly allergic, you may experience a very intense reaction upon a food's reintroduction. If you have been very reactive to certain foods in the past, I recommend that you check with your physician before returning possible problem foods to your diet.

On the other hand, symptoms of allergy and other intolerances can be sporadic in nature. Some people are able to enjoy their "allergic foods" if they indulge only occasionally. If you notice any symptom reduction by eliminating a specific food but find that you can enjoy it occasionally without a flare-up, I strongly recommend that you eat the food no more frequently than every four days. Called a rotation diet, this strategy, which reduces the body's reactive load, can be helpful in controlling symptoms and preventing the development of more allergies.

Finally, if you suspect food allergies but are not able to pinpoint the offending substance, do not hesitate to seek help from a qualified physician who can perform tests to determine exactly what is causing the problem. (See the inset on page 45.)

A FINAL NOTE ABOUT PROBLEM FOODS

In Chapter 3, you learned about oxalate-rich foods—a group of foods that, in some people, can cause or worsen inflammatory conditions. If you do not get full benefits from the dietary protocols discussed earlier in this chapter, I suggest you adopt the low-oxalate diet discussed in Chapter 3. I do not, however, recommend trying to blend the anti-inflammatory diet outlined in this chapter with the low-oxalate diet. Because it would involve so many restrictions, such a diet would be too difficult to manage. Instead, if the restrictions discussed in this chapter do not prove useful, I suggest that you try following a low-oxalate diet alone.

AN ANTI-INFLAMMATORY LIFESTYLE

Often, lifestyle changes are harder to make than dietary changes. It is easy to toss a colorful salad for lunch, but it's difficult to find the time to relax and truly take care of yourself. Many of us work two jobs, juggling the responsibilities at work with the needs of our families. Our own needs get scribbled on the bottom of the to-do list—and we never get to the end of the page.

That is precisely what we must change if we are to bring the raging inflammation under control. We must practice self-care.

Coping With Stress

In Chapter 3, I discussed some of the studies which

show that emotional stress—especially anger, hostility, and depression—increases inflammation. Physical stress brought on by hard physical work and illness has also been proven to contribute to inflammatory conditions. You can see, then, how important it is to find ways to reduce the stress in your life.

Fortunately, there are many ways to cope with stress and improve your outlook. It may be as simple as making a little more time in your day for the things you love, whether that involves reading, gardening, taking a walk, watching movies, or spending more time with friends and loved ones. If you have been telling yourself that you don't have time to read a book or watch a movie, consider this a prescription to relax. It is usually cheaper than drugs, it has no side effects, and it often can do wonders for both your mental and physical health.

If friends and hobbies are not the answer to your stress, consider that help may be as close as your local library or bookstore. Many simple yet effective forms of relaxation techniques, from meditation to breathing exercises, can be learned in the privacy of your home with a little guidance from a book or tape. Just be aware that it may take some time before you begin to see the benefits of these techniques.

Finally, if you cannot find relief from stress on your own, don't hesitate to contact a health-care professional. A qualified professional can help you in a variety of ways—with biofeedback therapy, hypnotherapy, guided imagery training, and/or psychological counseling. Again, these therapies may take some time to work, but your body will thank you!

Getting Adequate Rest

The average American is sleep deprived by one and a quarter hours per night. And sleep deprivation has been shown to fuel inflammation.

If you had lived in the early 1800s, you would have been awakened by the sun, and begun your day of work only when it was light enough to see. And when the fading rays of light disappeared, you would have gone to bed. But thanks to Thomas Edison and the incandescent light bulb, we can now work twenty-four hours a day. We use the waning evening hours to do work that did not get done at the office. If we do not work twelve hours a day, we feel lazy.

Well, our bodies do not think as we do. They are tired most of the time, and they respond by sending out messages of inflammation that eat away at the heart and cause pain throughout the body. If we want to be healthy again, we simply must rest.

How can you get adequate sleep? To start, try to retire for the night by 10:00 PM, and relax before you turn out the light. Enjoy a romantic interlude with your spouse. Read a good book. Meditate or pray. Cuddle your kids. Sip a cup of chamomile tea. Knit.

Just as important, make a special effort to avoid activities that can be stimulating or upsetting. Do not watch television—especially the news—directly before retiring. TV can be overstimulating. Do not bring work to bed with you. Do not exercise vigorously just before retiring, as the adrenaline push stimulated by the workout can keep you awake. And do not get into an argument with a family member. Also avoid stimulating substances such as coffee, cocoa, and alcohol—

which should be avoided anyway because of their inflammatory effects. Note that although alcohol may temporarily make you feel sleepy, it can interfere with normal sleep cycles.

Finally, be sure your bedroom is well ventilated and completely dark so that your body will produce adequate amounts of the sleep hormone melatonin. Darkness is your body's signal to enjoy deep refreshing sleep.

A Prescription for Complete Rest

Although we all know the importance of adequate sleep and relaxation, the demands of everyday life often keep us from getting the rest we need. And most vacations actually make the situation worse as we run from activity to activity, trying to get the most out of our precious holiday.

What is the answer? Go on a twenty-four-hour silent retreat where you allow no sound or distractions at all. Check into a quiet bed-and-breakfast or motel. Visit the beach or the mountains. Go alone or with a friend, and make a pact of no communication. No TV. No radio. No cell phone. No computer. Spend the time sleeping, meditating, reading, taking relaxing walks, or just thinking in absolute silence.

After your brain finally gets the rest it needs—and it may take hours before it can quiet itself—you will experience an incredible sense of peace that restores the body and mind. Do it often. Your body will love it.

DOES YOUR BODY NEED REALIGNMENT?

Many years ago, I fell off a horse and landed on the small of my back. I was not seriously injured; my back hurt for a few weeks and after several rounds of good chiropractic treatment, I felt fine. But since that time, if I eat foods to which I am allergic or do not get enough rest, that part of my back hurts. And this has not been my experience alone. Studies have shown that people who have experienced physical injury are generally more prone to inflammatory problems.

Not just accidents, but also a sedentary lifestyle can lead to weakening of a body area and, ultimately, to inflammation. Our bodies were meant to move and work. We were not meant to sit for eight to twelve hours per day, in a chair that was not designed to fit the normal human frame. Yet many of us spend an hour or more in the car or train every morning, commuting to our workplace. We sit in front of a computer screen for eight or more hours, getting up only to go to lunch or attend to personal needs. We return to the car for the commute home, sit during dinner, sit in front of the TV screen, and walk only a few steps to go to bed. That type of activity pattern can wreak havoc on posture, throwing the spine—and subsequently, the rest of the body—out of its normal position. Once bones are misaligned, muscles must compensate to maintain the upright position, increasing the tendency of the body to further shift out of position. Gradually, wear and tear begins to erode the bone structure itself. Predictably, the result is inflammation.

What's the answer? Certainly, realignment of the spine through chiropractic care can provide much-

Exercise Is Anti-Inflammatory!

If you are considering ways to reduce inflammation, don't overlook one of the simplest and most common prescriptions of all—exercise. We all know that exercise is good for cardiovascular health. But did you know that exercise has also been proven to relieve inflammatory disease all over the body? Specifically, physical activity has been found to lower levels of several inflammatory markers, including C-reactive protein, fibrinogen, and factor A clotting activity. Of course, if you've been inactive for some time, you'll want to check with your physician before starting an exercise regimen.[4]

needed help. But don't overlook the importance of vigorous exercise, which allows the body to realign and normalize itself. Many people who, like me, suffered from some type of injury, have found that the pain of inflammation diminishes through physical activity.

Smart dietary and lifestyle changes can do a world of good, gradually dampening the fires of existing inflammation and preventing future flare-ups. But if you currently suffer from the pain of arthritis or another inflammatory condition, you probably want more immediate help. In Chapter 4, you learned the drawbacks of the various anti-inflammatory pharmaceuticals currently offered by conventional medicine. Are there any alternatives? Absolutely! In the next chapter, you will learn about the many natural anti-inflammatory products that can help your body heal—without the side effects associated with conventional drugs.

6

NATURAL
ANTI-INFLAMMATORIES

In Chapter 5, you learned of the many dietary and life-style changes that can remove anti-inflammatories from your life and help your body gradually regain and maintain a healthy state. But if arthritis or another inflammatory disorder is causing you pain and discomfort, you understandably want relief *fast*. While drugs can sometimes offer speedy relief, they often do so at a price—a price that can be as relatively small as stomach pain or as great as heart disease. Fortunately, there are a number of natural alternatives that are proven to be not only safe, but also truly effective in the war against inflammation. That is what this chapter is all about.

In the following pages, you will learn about a range of natural anti-inflammatories. Each discussion begins with background information about the substance so that you will know what it is and where it comes from. After that, you will read about the scientific studies that have proven its effectiveness. This is followed by information on safe usage, and, finally, by information on dosage.

Be aware that while the remedies explored in this chapter are generally very well tolerated, the power and potency of natural medicinals is very real. It is, therefore, important to know of possible side effects of a remedy before you take it. That's why the "Is It Safe?" section has been included in the discussion of each anti-inflammatory. Read these sections, paying attention to the cautions regarding possible interactions with drugs, possible allergic reactions, and the like. Then, when you begin taking a preparation, note how it makes you feel, and adjust the dosage accordingly. Don't exceed the recommended dose unless counseled to do so by your health-care provider. Couple the information presented in these pages with careful observation and good judgment, and you will soon be reaping the benefits of natural anti-inflammatories.

BROMELAIN

Derived from the pineapple plant, bromelain is the name of a group of enzymes discovered in 1957. Among its many actions, bromelain has been found to be a powerful anti-inflammatory and blood thinner. It is thought to work by breaking down fibrin, a blood-clotting protein that can hamper good circulation and prevent tissues from draining. When inflammation is reduced, pain is also reduced and healing can begin.

Because of its anti-inflammatory action, bromelain has been used to treat sprains, strains, and muscle aches and pains; to alleviate back pain; to relieve the chronic joint pain associated with arthritis; to reduce the pain and swelling of gout; to ease respiratory allergies; and to reduce the tissue swelling associated with carpal tunnel syndrome. Bromelain is often combined with the enzyme trypsin and the flavonoid rutin for the treatment of osteoarthritis.

The Science Behind It

Bromelain has been studied for many years. The research performed on this natural anti-inflammatory includes the following:

Seventy-three patients with symptomatic osteoarthritis of the knee were randomized to receive three weeks of treatment with an enzyme preparation that contained bromelain, trypsin, and rutin, or a NSAID medication. The results of both treatment protocols were equivalent; in other words, both the bromelain and the medication treatment groups received the same benefits in terms of pain, function, various laboratory parameters, and tolerability.[1]

In a rat study on inflammation, the administration of bromelain was found to decrease both PGE2 (pro-inflammatory prostaglandin 2) and substance P (hormonal pain messenger).[2]

Is It Safe?

Bromelain is generally considered safe, even at high doses. However, it has been known to cause disturbances of the gastrointestinal tract such as stomach pain and diarrhea. Moreover, it should be avoided by people who are allergic to pineapples. This supplement is for short-term use only.

Because this enzyme is a natural blood thinner, bromelain should not be used with any blood-thinning medications, as it may increase the drug's effect.

The Recommended Dose

The standard dosage of bromelain is 80 to 320 mg divided into two or three doses per day. Osteoarthritis patients may use a bromelain product that also contains 100 mg of rutin and 48 mg of trypsin for added effectiveness. Note, though, that in studies, as much as 500 mg of bromelain has been safely taken three times daily, for a total of 1,500 mg. Therefore, you may want to start with a low dose and, if necessary, increase it for greater effectiveness. Bromelain should be taken for eight to ten days only.

CAT'S CLAW

Cat's claw (*U. tomentosa*) is a large, high-climbing woody vine that derives its name from hook-like thorns that grow at the base of the plant's leaves. This vine grows profusely in the upper Amazon regions of Peru, Columbia, Ecuador, and other South American countries. For hundreds of years, cat's claw been used as a medicinal by the indigenous peoples of the Amazon rainforest.

Among its many properties, cat's claw has been found to be a powerful anti-inflammatory. Both studies and anecdotal evidence suggest that it is useful in the treatment of arthritis of all kinds, bursitis, allergies, and a host of other inflammatory disorders. Moreover, it has analgesic properties, and thus helps to relieve the pain of inflammation.

The Science Behind It

Cat's claw has been studied for many years. The

research performed on this natural anti-inflammatory includes the following:

Cat's claw hinders the production of PGE2 and tumor necrosis factor-alpha (TNF-alpha), both of which are inflammatory agents. Because cat's claw works in an anti-inflammatory capacity, it is used for both osteoarthritis and rheumatoid arthritis. According to one research project, "Cat's claw is an effective treatment for osteoarthritis. The species, *U. guianensis* and *U. tomentosa* are . . . effective antioxidants, but their anti-inflammatory properties may result from their ability to inhibit TNF-alpha and to a lesser extent PGE2 production."[3]

Is It Safe?

There have been no reports of toxicity when cat's claw is taken at recommended doses. However, high doses may cause diarrhea, bleeding gums, excessive bruising, and a drop in blood pressure.

Because of its blood pressure-lowering action, cat's claw should not be taken along with antihypertensive medication, as it can increase the action of the drug. Because it has documented anti-fertility properties, cat's claw should not be taken by anyone who is seeking to get pregnant or is already pregnant. Due to its blood-thinning properties, it should not be taken with blood-thinning drugs. The herb should also be avoided by anyone with autoimmune disorders such as lupus or multiple sclerosis, because it has been found to stimulate the immune system, and thus may cause flare-ups. Finally, cat's claw should not be used before or after an organ or tissue transplant.

The Recommended Dose

For osteoarthritis, the recommended dosage of cat's claw is 100 mg taken daily in divided doses. For rheumatoid arthritis, the recommended dosage is 60 mg taken daily in divided doses.

CURCUMIN

Curcumin is an extract of turmeric—a spice well known for imparting a golden color and distinctive flavor to Indian and Thai cuisine. Curcumin has a long history of use in Ayurvedic medicine, where it is valued as an anti-inflammatory. Modern interest in the extract began in 1971, when Indian scientists began to explore the reason for turmeric's anti-inflammatory properties. The extract curcumin appears to reduce the synthesis of pro-inflammatory leukotriene and to promote the breakdown of fibrin, the blood-clotting protein that can prevent the proper drainage of tissues.

Curcumin has been found to have substantial anti-inflammatory effects in the treatment of rheumatoid arthritis. It has been shown to improve the duration of morning stiffness, to shorten walking time, and to diminish joint swelling.

The Science Behind It

Curcumin has been studied for many years. The research performed on this natural anti-inflammatory includes the following:

Human studies confirm evidence of curcumin's anti-inflammatory activity. Inflammatory compounds that are inhibited by the use of the extract include

phospholipase, lipoxygenase, cyclooxygenase 2, leukotrienes, thromboxane, prostaglandins nitric oxide, and
others.[4]

A study on the effects of curcumin on the aging
brain reported that curcumin has both antioxidant
and anti-inflammatory activities. In a rat study com-
paring conventional NSAIDs (ibuprofen) and curcumin, dietary curcumin but not ibuprofen, suppressed
oxidative and other types of age-related damage. Curcumin also reduced memory deficits and oxidative
deposits. Researchers believe that curcumin may help
prevent Alzheimer's disease (inflammation may play a
role in the genesis of Alzheimer's disease).[5]

Aberrant arachidonic acid metabolism is involved
in the inflammatory and carcinogenic processes. Researchers investigated the effects of curcumin on the
release of arachidonic acid and its metabolites, and
found that curcumin inhibited the release of arachidonic acid and prohibited the formation of PGE2.[6]

Is It Safe?

A meta-analysis of curcumin that included studies on
the antioxidant, anti-inflammatory, antiviral, and anti-
fungal properties of the extract found no toxicity at
levels of up to 8,000 mg of curcumin per day when
taken for three months.[7] Reported side effects are
uncommon, and are limited to mild stomach distress.

The Recommended Dose

Standard recommended dosage for curcumin is 300 to
400 mg three times per day, or 4,000 to 40,000 mg of
turmeric—the whole spice—per day. Taking curcumin

with bromelain or fish oil may enhance absorption. If curcumin is used on its own, for maximum effectiveness, take on an empty stomach twenty minutes prior to each meal. When using the curcumin-fish oil combination, it is best to take the supplement with food. (Information on fish oil follows.)

FISH OIL

Fish oil is a rich source of the omega-3 fatty acids that have been found to have strong anti-inflammatory properties. Also known as fish body oil, omega-3 fatty acids, marine oils, PUFA (polyunsaturated fatty acids), and omega fatty acids, this important class of essential fats has been used to effectively reduce inflammation in the treatment of rheumatoid arthritis, Crohn's disease, ulcerative colitis, and a wide range of other inflammatory disorders.

Fish oils are believed to prevent and reduce inflammation by competing with arachidonic acid, a highly inflammatory substance, and thus inhibiting the production of a hormone that causes blood clotting and vasoconstriction. It should be noted that because of their potent anti-inflammatory actions, fish oils—besides being useful in the treatment of arthritis and other painful diseases—are also highly protective of cardiovascular health.

The Science Behind It

Fish oil has been studied for many years. The research performed on this natural anti-inflammatory includes the following:

Numerous clinical trials suggest that omega-3 fatty acids from fish oil are beneficial in the treatment of rheumatoid arthritis, psoriasis, asthma, and inflammatory bowel disorders. Given the evidence relating progression of atherosclerosis to chronic inflammation, the n-3 fatty acids may play an important role by damping down the inflammatory processes.[8]

In a review of 12 randomized, placebo-controlled, double-blind studies of rheumatoid arthritis, a daily dose of 2.6 g of fish oil resulted in improvement, including inhibiting the formation of specific immune complexes, reducing inflammation, and degrading enzymes. Reducing the amount of arachidonic acid (found in red meats) resulted in a further benefit from the fish oil.[9]

Is It Safe?

When standard doses of fish oil are used, there is no problem with toxicity. Good-quality supplements are virtually mercury-free. The most common side effect of this supplement is a fishy aftertaste. Other common reported side effects include gastrointestinal disturbances and nausea.

Because of the blood-thinning properties of this supplement, fish oil should not be taken when blood-thinning medications are also in use. If other cardiovascular medications are in use, it is wise to check with a nutritionally trained physician prior to using fish oil supplementation.

The Recommended Dose

The standard recommended dosage for fish oil is 1 to 4 g

per day, preferably taken with meals. Because oils are extremely volatile—sensitive to light, heat, and oxygen—it is imperative to select a high-quality product and to store it with care. First, look for the USP label on the supplement to insure that the oils do not contain harmful levels of contaminants. Do not buy fish oil supplements in bulk, but instead purchase enough for a few weeks only, preferably selecting a supplement packaged in a dark bottle to help prevent damage from light. Once the bottle is opened, store it in the refrigerator to protect it from heat, and use it up within a few weeks' time.

GINGER ROOT

Ginger was first used in China and India, and was introduced into Europe over 2,000 years ago. Although it is always referred to as a root, ginger is actually a rhizome—an underground stem of the tropical plant *Zingiber officinale.*

Ginger is a very versatile medicinal, and has been used by years to aid digestion and combat nausea. A lesser-known but equally potent action of ginger is to reduce inflammation—an effect that has been documented in several studies. It is thought that ginger's power as an anti-inflammatory may be due to an interruption of the prostaglandin-leukotriene cascade, which blocks the damaging (pro-inflammatory) prostaglandins but leaves the beneficial (anti-inflammatory) prostaglandins unaffected. Researchers have, in fact, compared ginger to the COX-2 inhibitors in its anti-inflammatory effects. It has also been found to inhibit platelet-activating factor (PAF), which is essential to the inflammatory process. Thus far, ginger has been used to alleviate headaches and the pain and inflammation of osteoarthritis and fibromyalgia.

The Science Behind It

Ginger has been studied for many years. The research performed on this natural anti-inflammatory includes the following:

A porcine study to determine the effects of an extract of ginger root on the production of nitric oxide (NO), a pro-inflammatory compound, and prostaglandin 2 (PGE2) found that exposing inflamed cartilage tissue to a preparation of ginger reduced the production of both inflammatory agents.[10]

Ginger may be particularly important for heart health—which, as we know, is linked to inflammation. An extract of ginger was used to determine the effect on serum cholesterol and triglycerides, as well as platelet thromboxane-B2 (a marker of inflammation) and PGE2. After four weeks of oral administration at a dosage level of 500 mg/kg, there was a significant reduction of serum PGE, thromboxane-B2, and serum cholesterol. There was no change in serum triglycerides.[11]

In an in vitro (test tube) study, ginger extract significantly inhibited the production and activation of two inflammatory compounds, TNF-alpha and COX-2, making it an appropriate anti-inflammatory herb, particularly in the treatment of arthritis.[12]

Is It Safe?

At prescribed dosage levels, ginger has no recorded

problems of significance, and no drug actions have been recorded. However, at high doses, ginger can cause heartburn and other gastrointestinal problems. Moreover, because of its blood-thinning properties and its other known effects, it is suggested that ginger may interfere with blood-thinning and other cardiac medications.

The Recommended Dose

The standard recommended dosage for ginger is 100 to 200 mg taken three times daily.

GLUCOSAMINE AND CHONDROITIN

Glucosamine and chondroitin are both natural substances found in the body. *Glucosamine* is an amino sugar—a compound consisting of an amino acid and a sugar molecule—that is synthesized by every cell in the body. It is found in particularly high concentrations in the cartilage and other connective tissues, and, among its many functions, it plays a role in the formation of cartilage. *Chondroitin sulfate* is part of a large protein molecule that gives cartilage its elasticity. It has been found to aid in preventing cartilage tissue from dehydrating and to assist in cushioning impact stress.

As we age, the body's ability to produce both glucosamine and chondroitin decreases, causing the wear and tear and hardening of cartilage associated with osteoarthritis. Supplements of glucosamine and chondroitin, which are extracted from animal tissue, have been found to support cartilage repair, thereby reducing both pain and inflammation. Many researchers have found that effectiveness is increased by using these products together.

The Science Behind It

Glucosamine and chondroitin have been studied for many years. The research performed on these natural anti-inflammatories includes the following:

In a study of 414 women with osteoarthritis of the knee, women taking 1,500 mg of glucosamine sulfate (GS) daily experienced no further loss in cartilage tissue, while the placebo group continued to experience cartilage destruction. The women taking the GS supplement also experienced a reduction in pain and an improvement in function.[13, 14, 15]

In a study of over 1,300 patients with osteoarthritis, those who took GS on a consistent basis enjoyed lower Osteoarthritis Index scores than those who took or used other products (NSAIDS, other pain medications, steroid injections, and mechanical aids).[16]

Studies of both glucosamine and chondroitin frequently show reduction in pain and improvement in function. However, the combination of the two components of the cartilage matrix, in supplement form, provides a synergistic effect, with a greater increase in the production of new cartilage tissue than either agent alone. The mechanisms of action are different for the products.[17]

Are They Safe?

So far, glucosamine and chondroitin have not been found to have serious side effects. The most common problems have been increased intestinal gas and loose stools. It has been suggested that switching brands can help to relieve these problems.

Because glucosamine is an amino sugar, however, it is thought that it may worsen insulin resistance, a major cause of diabetes. Therefore, people with diabetes should monitor their blood-sugar levels particularly carefully when using this supplement. There have been no reports of allergic reactions to glucosamine, but because this supplement is made from shellfish shells, people who are allergic to seafood should use it with caution or avoid it entirely.

Because chondroitin has blood-thinning effects, people who have bleeding disorders or are taking aspirin or blood-thinning medications should have their blood-clotting times checked.

The Recommended Doses

The standard recommended dosage for these supplements is 1,500 mg of glucosamine and 1,200 mg of chondroitin per day, divided into several doses.

MSM (METHYLSULFONYLMETHANE)

MSM, or methylsulfonylmethane, is a naturally occurring sulfur compound that is found in nearly all living organisms, and, not surprisingly, in many of our foods, including meat, fish, milk, eggs, legumes, nuts, fruits, vegetables, grains, and some algae. However, the processing and cooking of these products destroys or greatly reduces MSM content.

MSM was first discovered in the late 1970s by researchers at Oregon Health Sciences University in

Portland. Since then, research as shown that MSM is necessary for maintaining the health of connective tissue, cartilage, tendons, and ligaments, and that it lessens inflammation, inhibits pain impulses, and promotes joint mobility and comfort.

The Science Behind It

Several studies have been conducted on MSM's ability to reduce the pain of inflammation. The research performed on this natural anti-inflammatory includes the following:

After reports that MSM helped arthritis in animals, a double-blind, placebo-controlled study suggested that MSM, used either alone or in combination with glucosamine sulfate, is helpful in relieving the symptoms of knee osteoarthritis.[18]

Following this initial study, a double-blind clinical study examined the effectiveness of MSM for the treatment of osteoarthritis of the knee. In the study, 25 patients took MSM and 25 took a placebo for twelve weeks. Patients taking MSM were found to have significantly reduced pain and improved physical functioning, without major adverse effects. [19]

Is It Safe?

MSM is believed to be one of the least toxic substances in biology. It should be noted that the naturally occurring sulfur found in MSM is not similar to the inorganic sulfides, sulfites, and sulfates to which many people are allergic. However, it should also be noted that there are no peer-reviewed data on the effects of long-term use of MSM in humans.

The Recommended Dose

The standard recommended dose for this supplement is 1,000 to 3,000 mg per day, taken with meals. Some suggest that dosage should depend on body weight, with a 400-mg dose per every 50 pounds of weight.

ESSENTIAL MINERALS

Every cell in the body depends on minerals. Minerals are needed for the proper composition of body fluids, the formation of blood and bone, the maintenance of healthy nerve function, and the regulation of muscle tone. Minerals are considered coenzymes, which means that they enable the body to perform all of its many functions—including all functions relating to the control of inflammation.

Minerals also play an important antioxidant role, relieving the body of another causal factor in inflammation—oxidative stress. Several minerals also work to control inflammation by directly helping the body to fight acidity—a condition that, as you learned earlier in the book, sets the stage for inflammation.

The body is not able to produce a single mineral, but relies on outside sources for all of its mineral needs. While, ideally, the diet should supply the body with these important nutrients, mineral depletion in our soil makes our foods mineral-poor. Moreover, acidifying foods often rob the body of its minerals by causing it to draw upon mineral stores as a means of reducing acidity. It is critical, then, that you supplement your diet with the minerals it needs to function properly.

The Importance of Macro- and Micro-Minerals

All minerals are essential for good health. They help regulate and facilitate basic functions of the body, including energy production, growth, and healing. Minerals play an important role in the development of healthy bones, teeth, hair, and nails; they are also involved in proper nerve activity, muscle function, blood formation, and the regulation of hormones and bodily fluids.

Minerals are grouped into two categories—macrominerals and micro-minerals. Macro-minerals include calcium, magnesium, and phosphorus, and are needed by the body in dosages exceeding 100 milligrams per day. Minerals needed in much smaller amounts are considered micro-minerals, also called trace minerals. They include boron, chromium, copper, iodine, iron, manganese, potassium, selenium, silica, and zinc.

Because minerals are excreted from the body daily, they must be replaced in order to maintain optimum bodily functioning. While it is true that minerals are present in foods, and ideally a well-balanced and healthy diet should satisfy the body's need for them, our plants and soil have become nutrient depleted. Even eating the healthiest foods will not guarantee adequate mineral intake. For this reason, mineral supplementation is necessary. Macro-minerals are needed in larger amounts than micro-minerals. Although micro-minerals are required in minute quantities, they are still critical for optimum health.

The most important minerals in regard to controlling inflammation are boron, calcium, copper, magnesium, manganese, silica, and zinc. Let's learn about each of these important nutrients.

BORON

Recent studies have suggested that boron may play a role in preventing bone-related diseases such as osteoarthritis, rheumatoid arthritis, and osteoporosis. Boron is also important to the body's acid-alkaline balance because it enables the body to metabolize and make use of various other nutrients that work to maintain healthy pH levels and prevent inflammation.

The Science Behind It

Boron has been studied for many years. The research performed on this mineral includes the following:

In the case of osteo- and rheumatoid arthritis, scientists have found that boron can help improve patient symptoms.[20]

Studies have shown that there is an inverse relationship between the intake of boron and the incidence of arthritis.[21]

Is It Safe?

No health or medical problems associated with the use of boron have been reported in areas of the world where the daily diet supplies up to 41 mg per day of the mineral.

The Recommended Dose

Dosages of boron used in clinical studies range from

<1 mg to 10 mg daily, with the most common being 3 mg daily.

CALCIUM

Calcium is one of the primary acid-buffering minerals called upon by your body whenever excess acids pose a problem. The consequent depletion of calcium can be dangerous, as calcium is essential for the formation and maintenance of strong bones and teeth, as well as to regulate cardiovascular function, cell division, and muscle and nerve function. Thus, supplementation of this mineral is important to keep the body strong and resistant to a variety of disorders, and to help maintain the slightly alkaline environment that fights inflammation.

The Science Behind It

Calcium has been studied for many years. The scientific research performed on this mineral includes the following:

Calcium is commonly known for its role in the development and long-term health of bones and teeth.[22, 23] Calcium has also received much attention for its role in supporting bone health in postmenopausal women. Research suggests that calcium can slow, but not completely stop, the progression of osteoporosis. The body's need for calcium is greatest during periods of rapid growth, including childhood, pregnancy, and lactation.[24, 25]

Calcium may initiate muscle contractions. For this reason, it plays a vital role in maintaining a healthy heartbeat. It is also involved in the blood-clotting process. On the cellular level, calcium regulates the passage of nutrients and wastes through cell membranes. It is also involved in the regulation of various enzymes that control muscle contraction, fat digestion, and metabolism. Finally, calcium regulates the transmission of nerve impulses.

Is It Safe?

Calcium has been found safe at recommended dosage levels. However, people who have a history of kidney stones should consult their physician regarding calcium supplementation.

The Recommended Dose

The recommended calcium dosage level ranges from 500 to 2,000 mg daily.

COPPER

Copper is one of the building blocks of collagen and elastin, the proteins that provide structural integrity and elasticity for tissues, organs, and bones. It should not be surprising, then, that drugs containing copper complexes have been shown to be effective in combating many inflammatory diseases, including rheumatoid arthritis, osteoarthritis, ankylosing spondylitis, rheumatic fever, and sciatica. It is thought that the drugs' positive effects are due to copper's ability to facilitate or promote tissue repair processes that use copper-dependent enzymes.

Copper is also required for the production and function of hemoglobin, which is responsible for transporting oxygen throughout the body.

The Science Behind It

Copper has been studied for many years. The research performed on this mineral includes the following:

Targeted clinical applications for copper include its use as an aid in the prevention of osteoporosis and as an anti-inflammatory treatment for rheumatoid arthritis.[26, 27, 28]

Copper is also a component of two important enzymes. One is copper-containing superoxide dismutase (SOD), which is an important antioxidant. The other (dopamine beta-hydroxylase) is an enzyme that helps regulate the metabolism of vitamin C and the synthesis of the neurotransmitter norepinephrine.

Is It Safe?

In most cases, copper has been found safe at recommended dosage levels. However, in Wilson's disease, a rare hereditary disorder, copper accumulates in the liver or brain, causing toxicity. The symptoms of this condition can include hepatitis, degeneration of the lens of the eye, kidney malfunction, and neurological disorders. The disease is fatal if not diagnosed and properly treated.

The Recommended Dose

The recommended copper dosage level ranges from 0.5 to 2 mg daily.

MAGNESIUM

Magnesium is involved in more than 300 enzyme reactions in the body, including, of course, the reactions that help control inflammation. As a key player in calcium metabolism, magnesium is also important for the health and development of strong bones and teeth, thus making the body less vulnerable to hypocalcemia (low levels of calcium), osteoporosis, and arthritis. Finally, magnesium is a vital mineral for cardiovascular health, and is necessary for the transmission of nerve impulses, temperature regulation, detoxification, and energy production.

The Science Behind It

Magnesium has been studied for many years. The scientific research performed on this mineral includes the following:

Severe magnesium deficiency is linked to a pro-inflammatory response and increases in oxidative stress, but studies verify that even milder magnesium deficiency increases inflammation.[29]

Low levels of calcium are caused by deficiencies of both magnesium and calcium. Consequently, magnesium supplementation is as important as calcium supplementation. Low bone mass is a common feature of this condition. This may lead to osteoporosis and possibly other bone-related disorders. Studies also indicate that replacing lost calcium increases bone density in these patients, and that additional magnesium supplementation produces a further increase in bone mineral density.[30]

Magnesium deficiency is also associated with inflammatory bowel disease.[31] Supplementation is recommended, and for those who do not respond to oral supplementation, a daily intravenous dose of 200 to 400 mg of elemental magnesium is recommended.

Is It Safe?

In most cases, magnesium has been found safe at recommended dosage levels. Large doses of this dietary supplement, however, may result in diarrhea, and it may be necessary to lower the amount taken. Moreover, if you have kidney disease, you should talk to your doctor before taking this dietary supplement.

The Recommended Dose

The recommended range of magnesium is 400 to 1,000 mg per day. I recommend the citrate form, or a form that is blended with Kreb Cycle metabolites (alpha-ketoglutarate, aspartate, or taurinate). Both of these supplements are well absorbed.

MANGANESE

Although present in only trace amounts in body tissues, manganese is important for the healthy growth and maintenance of the body. Most important to those who are suffering from inflammation, manganese plays a critical role in the development and repair of tissues, cartilage, and bones—all structures that, when not adequately supported by nutrients, are vulnerable to inflammatory conditions.

The Science Behind It

Manganese has been studied for many years. The sci-

SierraSil—A Unique Mineral Supplement

Recently, a new mineral supplement emerged on the market, providing a unique combination of vital nutrients. This product has been shown to relieve arthritic pain and reduce inflammation.

SierraSil, a supplement containing minerals from a deposit found in the High Sierras, is comprised of numerous naturally occurring macro and trace minerals, including silica, calcium, potassium, magnesium, copper, iron, zinc, phosphorous, manganese, selenium, vanadium, chromium, boron, and molybdenum in a form that possesses unusual health-promoting properties.

SierraSil supplement was recently evaluated in an independent mechanism of action study conducted by Mark Miller, PhD, Professor of Cardiovascular Sciences at Albany Medical College.[32] Dr. Miller discovered that the supplement, when used either alone or in combination with an extract of cat's claw, significantly inhibits the deterioration of cartilage associated with both rheumatoid and osteoarthritis, and greatly reduces inflammation. Data from the study showed that in cultured human cartilage cells, SierraSil was able to significantly reduce the release of glycosaminoglycan and nitric oxide, which are both markers for the breakdown of cartilage.

In human clinical studies, 10 patients with previously diagnosed osteoarthritis of the knee were given either 2 grams of SierraSil, or SierraSil plus cat's claw extract. All patients experienced significant relief of pain, stiffness, and inflammation, as well as increased range of motion and stair-climbing ability, within one week of starting treatment, with no reported side effects.

Based upon the success of the small pilot study, a double-blind placebo controlled, multi-center study involving more than 100 patients was recently completed. Results again indicated that the patients experienced improved flexibility and quality of life.

Safety studies on SierraSil have included a LD50 (the lethal dose needed to kill 50 percent of the test population) study, in which animals were provided with doses of up to 80 times the recommended amounts. This resulted in increased body weight, improved overall health, and no mortalities. Sub-acute toxicity studies showed similar results.[33]

In this chapter, you learned the importance of minerals in the fight against inflammatory disease. This supplement—a natural blend of important minerals—appears to offer an effective and safe option for those suffering from arthritis and joint pain. (For more information on SierraSil, visit www.sierrasil.com.)

entific research performed on this mineral includes the following:

In addition to playing roles in the development and maintenance of tissues, cartilage, and bones, manganese is important in the regulation of blood clotting, supports the production of certain hormones and neurotransmitters, and assists in fat metabolism.

Research indicates that manganese supplementation may support health in diabetics, lower the frequency of seizures in people with epilepsy, help build strong bones, and also strengthen bones in patients with osteoporosis.[34, 35]

Is It Safe?

Manganese has been found safe at recommended dosage levels.

The Recommended Dose

The recommended dosage range for manganese is 250 mcg to 5 mg daily.

SILICA

The mineral silica is found in all tissues, and thus takes part in a wide range of body functions. This mineral is especially vital for the health of bones and cartilage. Swelling of the joints—including the swelling present in the inflammatory disease gout—is often a sign of silica deficiency.

The Science Behind It

Silica has been studied for many years. The research performed on this mineral includes the following:

Studies suggest that silica plays a role in the production of collagen; helps build healthy bones, teeth, and cartilage; may be associated with a decreased risk of atherosclerosis; may prevent and treat osteoporosis;[36, 37] and may stimulate the immune system.[38]

Research conducted by Dr. A. Charnot indicated

that silica supports the building of healthy bones. Animals kept on high silica diets attained maximal bone mineralization much quicker than did those on low-silica diets. As early as 1986, Edith M. Carlisle, PhD verified silica's role in connective tissue formation, noting that silica is a structural component of glycosaminoglycans (hyaluronic acids, chondroitin sulfates, and keratin sulphate) and their glycoprotein complexes. Carlisle noted that with the departure of silica from the interior (intimae) of artery walls and with the weakening of its connective tissue, comes a greater risk of developing occlusive heart disease.

Is It Safe?

Silica has been found safe and nontoxic at recommended dosage levels.

The Recommended Dose

The standard recommended dosage of silica is 20 to 40 mg daily.

ZINC

The mineral zinc is an essential component of over twenty enzymes associated with many different metabolic processes, including the antioxidant activities that help prevent inflammation. Perhaps most important, zinc is a vital part of the immune system—the system that controls the inflammatory response. It should not be surprising, then, that zinc appears to have anti-inflammatory properties.

The Science Behind It

Zinc been studied for many years. The research performed on this mineral includes the following:

Zinc helps regulate a wide variety of immune system functions and may stimulate antiviral activity and treat the common cold. Zinc has been studied for use in a wide range of other disorders and may have anti-inflammatory properties that could benefit arthritis sufferers.[39, 40, 41]

Is It Safe?

Recommended doses of zinc are safe, but regular intake greater than 150 mg per day could be a problem. Zinc toxicity can cause diarrhea, dizziness, drowsiness, lethargy, vomiting, and loss of muscle coordination. Tell your doctor if any of these effects occur.

The Recommended Dose

The standard recommended dosage of zinc is 25 to 50 mg daily.

This chapter has presented information on a number of products that have been proven both safe and effective. Used in combination with a diet of nutritious foods and other important lifestyle elements discussed in earlier chapters, these natural anti-inflammatories can start you on the road to a healthy pain-free life.

CONCLUSION

Despite the well-publicized problems associated with anti-inflammatory drugs, many people still resist trying natural anti-inflammatories. For them, the question remains: Do natural remedies really work?

In recent years, a growing body of science has validated the healing properties of foods, herbs, and other natural anti-inflammatories. However, as a health professional, I would be remiss if I did not tell you that some studies have reached different conclusions. While I may not agree with these results for a variety of scientific-based reasons, I try to keep an open mind to all serious research and discussion. But to really understand the power of natural healing, you have to experience it yourself. After using a natural remedy consistently, see if you find that you have less stiffness and less pain—that you can more comfortably perform daily tasks. If so, the scientists may refer to this as "anecdotal evidence." But for you, it will be relief!

Unfortunately, not everyone responds to natural remedies. Just as some people have derived relief from NSAIDs and others have not, some people simply don't respond to certain natural anti-inflammatories. And no one knows exactly why.

Perhaps the most important question to ask is: Will *you* respond to a natural approach to healing inflammation? It's easy to find out. This book was designed to start you on the road to drug-free relief. It may initially take a little work, but by choosing the right foods, reducing your stress, getting a good night's sleep, and using safe and natural remedies, you may find that you have not only reduced your pain and inflammation, but also regained a wonderful sense of health and well-being.

Enjoy life!

MENU PLAN
AND RECIPES

As discussed throughout this book, the journey to health starts in your kitchen. The following sample menu plan and recipes will help you understand how an anti-inflammatory diet is constructed. By using this plan, you will learn how to expand on a simple four-day rotation diet to include your favorite recipes *without* the inflammatory foods that may have contributed to your pain in the first place.

As you create your own anti-inflammatory menus, always keep in mind the dietary guidelines presented in Chapter 5. Eat lots of fresh fruits and vegetables; they are the cornerstone of the anti-inflammatory diet. Eliminate beef and pork; avoid the most common allergens—wheat, corn, and dairy; and include only modest portions of anti-inflammatory grains like brown rice, spelt, quinoa, millet, kamut, and amaranth. Also, rotate the proteins you eat—do not consume the same protein foods more frequently than once every four days. This will help you reduce the risk of developing food sensitivities. Finally, determine which, if any, of the nightshade vegetables and oxalate-rich foods—all discussed in Chapter 3—may be contributing to your inflammatory condition, and eliminate them from your diet as necessary. Many people have no problem with these foods, which is why I included tomatoes and potatoes—both nightshades—in some of the following recipes. But if these foods are reactive for you, avoid them or eat them only occasionally.

On the whole, the following dietary plan should greatly reduce food-induced inflammation. By following it, you should quickly begin to experience less pain and stiffness; your body will begin to heal.

FOUR-DAY ANTI-INFLAMMATORY MENU

Day One

Breakfast: Northwest Salmon Hash (page 87).

Lunch: Large bowl of Multi-Bean Soup (page 88), rice crackers, fresh fruit of your choice.

Dinner: Salmon Poached in White Wine (page 96), Vegetable Risotto (page 97), crudités (raw vegetables), Roasted Asparagus (page 95).

Snack: Fresh fruit or raw nut mix.

Day Two

Breakfast: Rice-based protein drink blended with fresh fruit and flax seed or olive oil.

Lunch: Curried Chickpeas and Kale (page 91), spelt bread.

Dinner: Braised Lamb (page 92), mashed potatoes, steamed carrots and peas.

Snack: Fresh fruit.

Day Three

Breakfast: 2 poached or fried eggs, 2 slices gluten-free bread (millet is good).

Lunch: Roasted Red Pepper Hummus (page 90) with rice crackers and fresh vegetables.

Dinner: Your favorite rotisserie or roasted chicken, baked sweet potatoes, large salad with several colorful vegetables topped with olive oil and a splash of balsamic vinegar.

Snack: Fresh fruit or raw nut mix.

Day Four

Breakfast: Brown Rice with Fruit and Nuts (page 86).

Lunch: A Salad You Could Enjoy Every Day (page 89).

Dinner: Southeast Asian Seafood Stew (page 94) over quinoa or rice.

Snack: Half avocado with a splash of olive oil and balsamic vinegar.

RECIPES

BROWN RICE WITH FRUIT AND NUTS

*You can actually start preparing the rice for this
breakfast dish the night before. Bring the water and salt
to boil in a small pot and stir in the rice. Cover tightly
and turn off the heat. By morning, the rice will be
nearly done. You'll need only to add a little
water and simmer the rice a few minutes.*

SERVES 2

$1\frac{1}{2}$ cups water

$\frac{1}{2}$ teaspoon salt

$\frac{3}{4}$ cup brown rice

1–2 cups diced fresh or frozen fruit,
such as strawberries, blueberries, and raspberries

1 cup walnuts or pecans

1. Bring the water and salt to boil in a small pot and stir
   in the rice. Reduce the heat to low, and simmer with
   the lid slightly ajar for 40 minutes, or until the water
   is absorbed and the rice is tender.

2. While the rice simmers, place the nuts in a small un-
   oiled skillet over medium-low heat. Stirring often,
   dry-roast the nuts 1 to 2 minutes, or until they begin
   to brown and turn fragrant. Be careful not to burn.
   Transfer the roasted nuts to a plate and let cool.

3. Add the fruit and nuts to the cooked rice and gently
   stir. Serve immediately.

NORTHWEST SALMON HASH

This easy-to-prepare dish is delightful for a leisurely weekend breakfast. Instead of salmon, feel free to use lamb or chicken for variety (leftovers are perfect), or dress it up with some fresh herbs.

SERVES 2

1 tablespoon olive oil

1 tablespoon butter

1 large baked potato, finely chopped

$\frac{1}{2}$ cup onion, diced

$\frac{1}{4}$ cup green bell pepper, diced

$\frac{1}{4}$ cup red bell pepper, diced

1 clove garlic, minced

3–4 ounces cooked salmon

1. Heat the olive oil and butter in a large frying pan (an iron skillet works best) over medium heat.

2. Add the potato, onion, green and red bell peppers, and garlic. Sauté until the potatoes are lightly browned on the bottom. Turn the mixture over and brown the other side, stirring occasionally to prevent burning.

3. When the vegetables are nearly cooked, break up the salmon and add it to the frying pan. When the salmon is warm and the potatoes are browned, serve immediately.

MULTI-BEAN SOUP

*Although you can gather your own assortment of beans
for this soup, you can also buy them already packaged at
your local health food store (brands such as Bob's Red
Mill make it easy for you). One thing is certain—this
soup is delicious, no matter where you get the beans!*

SERVES 8 TO 10

2 cups mixed dried beans (such as navy, black,
red, pinto, baby limas, large limas, Great Northern,
kidney, chickpeas, black-eyed peas, yellow
split peas, green split peas, and lentils)

1 cup chopped onion

2 cloves garlic, minced

15-ounce can tomato sauce,
or 4 cups chopped tomatoes

1 teaspoon chili powder, or to taste

1. Rinse the beans, cover with fresh water, and let soak
   overnight.

2. Drain and rinse the soaked beans, then place in a
   large pot with $2\frac{1}{2}$ quarts fresh water. Bring to a boil,
   then reduce the heat to low and simmer covered
   3 to $3\frac{1}{2}$ hours, or until the beans are tender. Add the
   onion, garlic, tomato sauce, and chili powder, and
   simmer another 30 minutes.

3. Serve hot.

A SALAD YOU COULD ENJOY EVERY DAY

*I can have this salad on the table, beautifully arranged,
within fifteen minutes. Not only is it attractive, it is
sensationally delicious. I sometimes use shrimp or
crabmeat instead of snapper, but feel free to vary this
recipe according to your own likes or dislikes.*

SERVES 2

1 tablespoon butter and olive oil mixture

2 snapper or other fish filets (3 to 4 ounces each)

6 cups mesclun or mixed dark lettuce varieties

1 cup grape or cherry tomatoes

1 small cucumber, peeled and cut into $\frac{1}{4}$-inch slices

1 cup dried cranberries or cherries

1 cup raw pecans, walnuts, or other nut

$\frac{1}{4}$ cup chèvre or other soft goat cheese, such as feta

1. Heat the butter-olive oil mixture in a small skillet
   over medium-high heat. Add the fish and cook about
   3 minutes on each side, or until cooked through.

2. While the fish cooks, assemble the lettuce, tomatoes,
   cucumber, cranberries, nuts, and chèvre on two plates.
   Sprinkle with your favorite dressing.

3. As soon as the fish is cooked, place one filet on top of
   each salad and serve.

ROASTED RED PEPPER HUMMUS

This hummus is absolutely delicious and very easy to prepare. You can vary this recipe by replacing the red peppers with other flavorful ingredients, such as pesto or roasted garlic.

SERVES 4

2 cans (16 ounces each) chickpeas

1–2 large roasted red peppers

1 cup tahini

2 tablespoons lemon juice

5 cloves garlic

1. Drain the chickpeas, reserving the liquid.

2. Place all of the ingredients in a food processor, including a little of the reserved chickpea liquid. Purée until smooth, adding additional liquid as needed to achieve the desired consistency.

3. Refrigerate a few hours to allow the flavors to blend. Let the hummus come to room temperature before serving.

CURRIED CHICKPEAS AND KALE

While this dish simmers gently in the crockpot,
its tantalizing aroma will entice everyone
(perhaps even the neighbors) to the kitchen.
Ladle the rich broth over rice, or sop it up
with a crust of whole grain gluten-free bread.

Serves 2 to 4

3 cups cooked chickpeas

3 cups chopped kale

1 $\frac{1}{2}$ cups chopped onions

1 $\frac{1}{2}$ cups chicken or vegetable broth

1 cup canned or fresh chopped tomatoes

4 cloves garlic, crushed

2 tablespoons olive oil

1 $\frac{1}{2}$ tablespoons curry powder

1 teaspoon ground ginger

1 teaspoon ground coriander

$\frac{1}{2}$ teaspoon cumin

$\frac{1}{4}$ teaspoon salt, optional

1. Place all of the ingredients in a crockpot. Cover and cook on high for 4 hours.

2. Enjoy plain as a stew or served over rice.

BRAISED LAMB

I love the way this lamb is prepared and make it often.
In addition to enjoying it as a main course,
I use it in shepherd's pie, add it to sandwiches,
and toss it in salads.

SERVES 6 TO 8

5 1/2-pound lamb shanks or shoulder

2 tablespoons olive oil

Salt to taste

Pepper to taste

2 small onions, quartered

1/2 cup fresh thyme sprigs

1/2 cup fresh rosemary sprigs

1 1/2 cups water

1 1/4 cups no-sodium beef broth

1/2 cup dry white wine

Gravy

2 1/2 cups cooking broth from the lamb

1 tablespoon corn or potato starch

1. Preheat the oven to 450°F.

2. Place the lamb in a large metal roasting pan. Rub with oil, season with salt and pepper, and surround with onion wedges.

3. Roast the lamb in middle of the oven for 40 minutes. Turn it over, scatter with thyme and rosemary, and continue to roast another 40 minutes.

4. Pour the water, broth, and wine into the pan, cover with a lid or foil, and continue to cook 45 to 60 minutes, or until the lamb is tender.

5. Transfer the lamb to a plate and set aside. Pour the cooking broth (including the onions) into a large glass measuring cup. Do not clean the pan.

6. To make the gravy, skim the fat from the cooking broth (there should be $2\frac{1}{2}$ cups of broth left). Pour 1 cup of the broth into a large bowl, add the starch, and whisk to form a thin paste. Whisk in the remaining broth.

7. Set the roasting pan on the stovetop across two burners. Pour the broth mixture into the pan and bring to a boil over medium heat, whisking constantly until thickened. Remove from the heat and season with salt and pepper.

8. Remove the lamb from the bone, cut into bite-sized pieces, and add to the roasting pan. Mix with the gravy, and serve.

SOUTHEAST ASIAN SEAFOOD STEW

*This savory crockpot dish is aromatic and delicious—
simply wonderful.*

SERVES 4

8 ounces fresh or frozen white fish, cut into chunks

3 medium tomatoes, cut into small wedges

1 medium onion, chopped

4 cloves garlic, minced

$\frac{1}{2}$ cup chopped fresh cilantro or parsley

8-ounce can tomato sauce

1 cup white wine

1 cup vegetable stock, no salt added

$\frac{1}{4}$ cup olive oil

$\frac{1}{4}$ cup fresh-squeezed lime juice

2 teaspoons grated fresh ginger

2 cups water

1 cup brown rice

5 ounces fresh prawns, peeled and deveined

5 ounces fresh scallops

8 ounces fresh mussels or clams (in the shells)

2 limes, cut into wedges

1. Place the white fish, tomatoes, onion, garlic, cilantro, tomato sauce, wine, stock, oil, lime juice, and ginger in a crockpot. Cover and cook on low heat for 6 to 8 hours.

2. About 40 minutes before serving, bring the water to boil in a small pot. Stir in the rice, cover, and simmer gently about 35 to 40 minutes, or until the rice is tender.

3. About 30 minutes before serving, add the prawns, scallops, and mussels to the crockpot, and continue to cook 30 minutes, or until the shellfish are cooked.

4. To serve, place a spoonful of rice in individual bowls and top with a generous portion of stew. Garnish with a lime wedge.

ROASTED ASPARAGUS

This recipe is so simple,
you'll likely find yourself making it often.

SERVES 4

1 pound fresh asparagus spears,
washed and trimmed

1 tablespoon olive oil

1. Preheat the oven to 350°F.

2. Place the asparagus in a baking dish and drizzle with oil. Bake uncovered 15 to 20 minutes, or until tender.

3. Serve hot.

SALMON POACHED IN WHITE WINE

*For added taste and eye appeal, top this simple dish
with a salsa made of finely chopped mango, avocado,
red onion, and splash of balsamic vinegar.
Beautiful and delicious!*

SERVES 2

1 tablespoon olive oil

2 salmon filets (3 to 4 ounces each)

$\frac{1}{2}$ cup dry white wine

Pinch salt

1. Heat the olive oil in a sauté pan over medium heat until it just begins to bubble.

2. Add the salmon and sauté 2 to 3 minutes on each side until lightly browned.

3. Add the wine, cover, and lower the heat slightly. Let the salmon steam for 3 to 4 minutes or until moist and slightly pink in the center.

4. Transfer the salmon to a plate, spoon the cooking sauce on top, and serve immediately.

VEGETABLE RISOTTO

*This is such a simple, delicious rice dish,
you'll want to enjoy it often.*

SERVES 4 TO 6

1 tablespoon olive oil

1 tablespoon butter

1–2 cups diced carrots, celery, onion,
and garlic combination

2 cups water

1 cup brown rice

1. Heat the olive oil and butter in a large heavy pot over medium heat.

2. Add the vegetables, and sauté 3 to 4 minutes, or until they begin to brown.

3. Stir the water and rice into the pot and bring to a boil. Reduce the heat to low, and simmer with the lid slightly ajar for 15 minutes, or until the water is absorbed and the rice is tender.

4. Season with salt and pepper, if desired, and serve.

ROASTED ROOT VEGETABLES

*This recipe works with any fresh root vegetable found in
the produce department of your supermarket. If you can
purchase organic varieties, even better! For an added
flavor boost, sprinkle a little balsamic vinegar over the
roasting vegetables near the end of cooking time.*

SERVES 4 TO 6

3 tablespoons olive oil

6 cups mixed root vegetables,
cut into 1-inch chunks (good choices
include turnips, daikon, and carrots)

2 tablespoons chopped fresh parsley

Salt to taste

Pepper to taste

1. Preheat the oven to 425°F.

2. Coat the bottom of a large roasting pan with the olive
   oil. Add the root vegetables, parsley, salt, and pepper,
   and stir to coat with oil.

3. Stirring the vegetables every 15 minutes, roast for
   about 1 hour, or until tender and nicely browned.

4. Serve hot.

LENTILS AND GREENS

This recipe was graciously provided by organic farmers
Chris and Eva Worden of Worden Farms
in Punta Gorda, Florida.

SERVES 2

2 tablespoons olive oil

1 clove garlic, minced

1 cup lentils

4 cups water

6 cups shredded kale or collards

1 carrot, sliced into rounds

1 tablespoon ground cumin

Salt to taste

Pepper to taste

1. Heat the oil in a medium-sized pot over medium heat. Add the garlic and sauté 1 or 2 minutes until fragrant and beginning to soften.

2. Stir the lentils and water into the pot, cover, and simmer gently for 15 minutes. Add the remaining ingredients, and continue to simmer 15 minutes or until the lentils are tender. Add additional water if needed.

3. Serve as is or spooned over rice.

RESOURCES

ORGANIZATIONS

The following organizations of physicians and health-care professionals support the research of alternative methods of medical treatment, and promote awareness of the latest findings in this area. They supply helpful information and provide referrals for local health-care providers, including nutritionists, naturopathic and holistic physicians, doctors of osteopathy, and/or medical doctors.

American College for Advancement in Medicine (ACAM)
23121 Verdugo Drive, Suite 204
Laguna Hills, CA 92653
PHONE: 949-583-7666 • 800-532-3688
FAX: 949-455-9679
EMAIL: info@acam.org
WEBSITE: www.acam.org
Medical society dedicated to educating physicians and other health-care professionals on the latest findings in preventive/nutritional medicine. Provides contacts of holistic, naturopathic, and medical physicians.

American Association of Naturopathic Physicians (AANP)

3201 New Mexico Avenue, NW - Suite 350
Washington, DC 20016
PHONE: 202-895-1392 • 866-538-2267
FAX: 202-274-1992
EMAIL: member.services@naturopathic.org
WEBSITE: www.naturopathic.org
National professional society of physicians who use natural healing protocols in their medical practice. Provides listing of naturopathic physicians.

International and American Associations of Clinical Nutritionists (IAACN)

15280 Addison Road, Suite 130
Addison, TX 75001
PHONE: 972-407-9089
FAX: 972-250-0233
EMAIL: dvestal@clinicalnutrition.com
WEBSITE: www.iaacn.org
Professional association of practicing clinical nutritionists in a variety of health-care professions. Offers referrals of certified nutritionists.

National Association of Nutrition Professionals (NANP)

PO Box 971
Veradale, WA 99037-0971
PHONE: 800-342-8037
FAX: 510-580-9429
WEBSITE: www.nanp.org

Association of nutrition professionals dedicated to promoting the continued advancement of knowledge in the field of nutrition. Provides referrals of certified nutritionists.

Vulvar Pain Foundation
203 ½ North Main Street, Suite 203
Graham, NC 27253
PHONE: 336-226-0704
FAX: 336-226-8518
WEBSITE: www.vulvarpainfoundation.org
Provides lists of foods that can and cannot be eaten on a low-oxalate diet (referred to in Chapter 3).

REFERENCES

Chapter 3. Fueling the Fire

1. Voilley, N; J de Weille; and J Mamet, et al. "Nonsteroid Anti-Inflammatory Drugs Inhibit Both the Activity and the Inflammation-Induced Expression of Acid-Sensing Ion Channels in Nociceptors." *J Neurosci* Oct 15, 2001; 21(20):8026–8033.

2. Suarez, E; S Wassertheil; and L Wulsin. *Psychosomatic Medicine* September 2004, Vol. 66.

3. Steeves, S. WebMD Medical News, March 12, 2001.

4. *Archives of General Psychiatry* October 2003, Vol. 60:00, 1009–1014.

5. Ladwig, K. *Brain, Behavior and Immunity* 2003, Vol. 17, 268–275.

Chapter 5. A Holistic Approach

1. Zampelas, A; and DB Panagiotakos, et al. "Associations Between Coffee Consumption and Inflammatory Markers in Healthy Persons: The ATTICA Study." *Am J Clin Nutr* 2004; 80:862–867.

2. Lopez-Garcia, E; MB Schulze; and TT Fung, et al. "Major Dietary Patterns Are Related to Plasma Concentrations of Markers of Inflammation and Endothelial Dysfunction." *Am J Clin Nutr* 2004; 80:1029–1035.

3. Janin, B. "Mediterranean Diet Associated With Fewer Cardiovascular Events." *Family Practice News* January 1, 2004.

4. Panagiotakos, DB; and P Kokkinos, et al. "Physical Activity and Markers of Inflammation and Thrombosis Related to Coronary Heart Disease." *Prev Cardiol* Fall 2004; 7:190–194.

Chapter 6. Natural Anti-Inflammatories

1. Klein, G; and W Kullich. "Short-Term Treatment of Painful Osteoarthritis of the Knee With Oral Enzymes." *W Clinical Drug Investigation* January 1, 2000.

2. Gaspani, L; E Limiroli; and P Rerrario, et al. "In Vivo and In Vitro Effects of Bromelain on PGE(2) and SP Concentrations in the Inflammatory Exudate in Rats." *Pharmacology* May 2002; 65(2):83–86.

3. Piscoya, J.; Z Rodriguez; and SA Bustamante, et al. "Efficacy and Safety of Freeze-Dried Cat's Claw in Osteoarthritis of the Knee: Mechanisms of Action of the Species Uncaria Guianensis." *Inflammation Research* 50 (2001) 442–448.

4. Chainani-Wu, N. "Safety and Anti-Inflammatory Activity of Curcumin: A Component of Turmeric (Curcuma longa)" *J Altern Complement Med* February 2003; 9(1): 161–168.

5. Frautschy, SA; W Hu; and P Kim, et al. "Phenolic Anti-Inflammatory Antioxidant Reversal of Abeta-Induced Cognitive Deficits and Neuropathology." *Neurobiol Aging* November–December 2001; 22(6):993–1005.

6. Hong, J; M Bose; and J Ju, et al. "Modulation of Arachidonic Acid Metabolism by Curcumin and Related Beta-Diketone Derivatives: Effects on Cytosolic Phospholipase A(2), Cyclooxygenases and 5-Lipoxygenase." *Carcinogenesis* September 2004; 25(9):1671–1679.

7. Chainani-Wu, N. "Safety and Anti-Inflammatory Activ-

ity of Curcumin: A Component of Turmeric (Curcuma longa)." *J Altern Complement Med* February 2003; 9(1): 161–168.

8. Mori, TA; and LJ Beilin."Omega-3 Fatty Acids and Inflammation." *J Curr Atheroscler Rep* November 2004; 6(6):461–467.

9. Adam, O. "Dietary Fatty Acids and Immune Reactions in Synovial Tissue." *Eur J Med Res* August 20, 2003; 8: 381–387.

10. Shen, CL; KJ Hong; and SW Kim."Effects of Ginger (Zingiber officinale Rosc.) on Decreasing the Production of Inflammatory Mediators in Sow Osteoarthritic Cartilage Explants." *J Med Food* Winter 2003; 6(4):323–328.

11. Thomson, M; KK Al-Qattan; and SM Al-Sawan, et al. "The Use of Ginger (Zingiber officinale Rosc.) as a Potential Anti-Inflammatory and Antithrombotic Agent." *Prostaglandins Leukot Essent Fatty Acids* December 2002; 67(6): 475–478.

12. "An In Vitro Screening Assay for Inhibitors of Proinflammatory Mediators in Herbal Extracts Using Human Synoviocyte Cultures." *In Vitro Cell Dev Biol Anim* March–April 2004; 40(3–4):95–101.

13. Bruyere, O. *Menopause* March–April 2004; Vol. 11: 138–143.

14. Pavelka, K. *Archives of Internal Medicine* October 14, 2002; Vol. 162: 2113–2123.

15. Reginster, JY. *The Lancet* January 27, 2001; Vol. 357: 251–256.

16. Kirn, TF. "Glucosamine Helps Osteoarthritis More Than Other Treatments, Study Finds." *Family Practice News* December 1, 2004:51.

17. Owens, S; P Wagner; and CT Vangsness. "Recent Advances in Glucosamine and Chondroitin Supplementation." *J Knee Surg* October 2004; 17(4):185–193.

18. Usha PR, Naidu MUR. Randomised, double-blind, parallel, placebo-controlled study of oral glucosamine, methylsulfonylmethane and their combination in osteoarthritis. *Clin Drug Invest* 2004; 24(6): 353—63.

19. Kim LS, Axelrod LJ, Howard P, Buratovich N, Waters RF. Efficacy of methylsulfonylmethane (MSM) in osteoarthritis pain of the knee: a pilot clinical trial. *Osteoarthritis Cartilage* 2006; 14(3): 286—94.

20. Travers, RL, et al. "Boron and Arthritis: The Results of a Double-Blind Study." *J Nutr Med* 1990; 1:127–132.

21. Newnham, RE. "Arthritis or Skeletal Fluorosis and Boron." *Int Clin Nutr Rev* 1991; 11(2): 68–70.

22. Abrams, SA. "Calcium Turnover and Nutrition Through the Life Cycle." *Proc Nutr Soc* May 2001; 60(2): 283–289.

23. O'Brien, KO; MS Nathanson; J Mancini; and FR Witter. "Calcium Absorption Is Significantly Higher in Adolescents During Pregnancy Than in the Early Postpartum Period." *Am J Clin Nutr* December 2003; 78(6):1188–1193.

24. Dawson-Hughes, B. "Calcium Supplementation and Bone Loss: A Review of Controlled Clinical Trials." *Am J Clin Nutr* July 1991; 54(1):274S–280S.

25. Wishart, JM; PM Clifton; and BE Nordin. "Effect of Perimenopause on Calcium Absorption: A Longitudinal Study." *Climacteric* June 2000; 3(2):102–108.

26. Strain, JJ. "A Reassessment of Diet and Osteoporosis— Possible Role for Copper." *Med Hypotheses* December 1988; 27(4):333–338.

27. Sorenson, JR, et al. "Treatment of Rheumatoid and Degenerative Diseases With Copper Complexes: A Review with Emphasis on Copper-Salicylate." *Inflammation* September 1997; 2(3): 217–238.

28. Klevay, LM. "Lack of a Recommended Dietary Allowance for Copper May Be Hazardous to Your Health." *J Am Coll Nutr* August 1998; 17(4): 322–326.

29. Kramer, JH; IT Mak; and TM Phillips, et al. "Dietary Magnesium Intake Influences Circulating Pro-Inflammatory Neuropeptide Levels and Loss of Myocardial Tolerance to Postischemic Stress." *Exp Biol Med* June 2003; 228(6):665–673.

30. Rude, RK; and M Olerich. "Magnesium Deficiency: Possible Role in Osteoporosis Associated With Gluten Sensitive Enteropathy." *Osteoporosis Int* 1996; 6:453–461.

31. Rosenberg, IH; JM Bengoa; and MD Sitrin. "Nutritional Aspects of Inflammatory Bowel Disease." *Ann Rev Nutr* 1985; 5:463–484.

32. Miller, M; and S Ahmed, et al. "Suppression of Human Cartilage Degradation and Chondrocyte Activation by a Unique Mineral Supplement SierraSil and a Cat's Claw Extract, Vincaria." *JANA* Vol. 7. No. 2:32–39.

33. Lieberman, Shari; and Alan Xenakis. *Mineral Miracle: Stopping Cartilage Loss & Inflammation Naturally.* Garden City Park, NY: Square One Publishers, 2006.

34. Freeland-Graves, J. "Manganese: An Essential Nutrient for Humans." *Nutrition Today* December 1988: 13–19.

35. Keen, CL, et al. "Nutritional Aspects of Manganese From Experimental Studies." *Neurotoxicology* April 1993; 20(2–3):213–223.

36. Eisinger, J, et al. "Effects of Silicon, Fluoride, Etidronate

and Magnesium on Bone Mineral Density: A Retrospective Study." *Magnes Res* September 1993; 6(3): 247–249.

37. Chapuy, MC, et al. "Prevention and Treatment of Osteoporosis." *Aging* (Milano) August 1995; 7(4):164–173.

38. Schiano, A, et al. "Silicon, Bone Tissue and Immunity." *Rev Rhum Mal Osteoartic* September 1979; 46(7–9):483–486.

39. Simkin, PA. "Oral Zinc Sulphate in Rheumatoid Arthritis." *Lancet* September 1976; 2 (7985):539–542.

40. Peretz, A, et al. "Effects of Zinc Supplementation on the Phagocytic Functions of Polymorphonuclears in Patients with Inflammatory Rheumatic Diseases." *J Trace Elem Electrolytes Health Dis* December 1994; 8(3–4): 189–194.

41. Cerhan, JR; KG Saag; LA Merlino; TR Mikuls; and LA Criswell. "Antioxidant Micronutrients and Risk of Rheumatoid Arthritis in a Cohort of Older Women." *Am J Epidemiol* February 2003; 157(4):345–354.

ABOUT THE AUTHOR

Carol Simontacchi, CCN, MS, is a certified clinical nutritionist and the author of a number of books on nutrition, including *Your Fat Is Not Your Fault, The Crazy Makers,* and *A Woman's Guide to a Healthy Heart.* She is a contributing writer for the *Healthy Hearts* newsletter, published online on eDiets.com, as well as the author and designer of *WINGS: Weight Success for a Lifetime*—a holistic weight-management curriculum.

Carol obtained her certification as a clinical nutritionist through the Clinical Nutritionist Certification Board. She is also a professional member of the International and American Associations of Clinical Nutritionists. She has served on the Education Committee of the National Nutritional Foods Association, and has served as the President of the Society of Certified Nutritionists.

Ms. Simontacchi, a highly sought-after lecturer, has appeared on numerous national, regional, and local radio and TV shows. Her work has been featured in *Newsday, First for Women, Woman's Day,* and other popular publications. Ms. Simontacchi currently lives with her family in Florida.

To learn more about Carol Simontacchi, including her ongoing weight- and health-management programs, visit her website at *www.islandnutritioncenter.meta-ehealth.com.*

INDEX